Pollution

and

Cancer:

a

toxic relationship

LEONARD HEALWISE

Table of contents

« *Pollution is the silent ghost in our air, water and soil; an insidious killer that lurks in the shadows of our daily lives, quietly sowing the seeds of cancer.* »

Introduction

Why this Book?

Why this book? The question is worth asking, because at its heart lies an issue that affects us all, in one way or another. In a world where industrial and technological progress has often taken precedence over the preservation of our environment, we are faced with a worrying reality: pollution, in its many forms, has become a constant companion in our daily lives. Its deleterious effects on our health are no longer in question, and among them, the link with the increase in cancer cases is increasingly obvious.

This book is therefore intended as a wake-up call, but also as a source of information and awareness-raising. It is not simply a collection of facts and scientific data; it is a mirror reflecting the stories of those who live day by day in polluted environments, and the accounts of those who have seen cancer knocking mercilessly at their door or that of their loved ones.

In these pages, we explore not only the scientific aspects of cancer and the various forms of pollution, but also delve into the human stories, struggles and hopes of those on the front line. This book attempts to build a bridge between the rigour of scientific research and the reality experienced by millions of people. It aims to show that behind every statistic there are faces, names and families.

The aim of this work is twofold. Firstly, to provide a clear and accessible understanding of the mechanisms by which pollution influences the development of cancer, based on the latest research in the field. Secondly, to give a voice to those whose lives have been shaped by this reality, by sharing their experiences, their challenges and their hopes.

This book is an invitation to look beyond the figures and studies. It is a call to recognise and understand the urgent need to act against pollution, not only as an environmental crisis, but also as a health crisis. It is a call for collective awareness, mobilisation and action to protect our health, the health of our loved ones and the health of future generations.

Ultimately, this book is not just another book about pollution and cancer. It is a testimony, a guide and a call to action. It represents a step towards a future where health and the environment are no longer in conflict, but coexist in harmony.

What we know on Cancer and Pollution

What we know about cancer and pollution is a body of facts and knowledge that has been built up over the years, through rigorous studies, in-depth research and field observations. This is an area where science meets the day-to-day reality of individuals, revealing a picture that is both complex and alarming.

Cancer, this multifaceted and often merciless disease, has long been regarded as a fatality, an inescapable consequence of genetics or ageing. However, our understanding has evolved. We now know that environmental factors, and pollution in particular, play a crucial role in the development of many types of cancer.

Pollution, whether in the air, water or soil, is not a visible enemy. It creeps into our environment in various forms: fine particles in the air we breathe, chemical contaminants in the water we drink, and toxic residues in the soil on which we live and grow our food. These pollutants are silent but frighteningly effective agents, capable of altering our biology at the most fundamental level, damaging DNA and disrupting cellular processes, creating a breeding ground for the development of cancer.
Epidemiological studies have established links between exposure to certain toxic substances and an increased risk of various cancers. For example, air pollution, classified as a human carcinogen by the World Health Organisation, has been linked to cancers of the lung, bladder and other organs. Contaminants in water, such as heavy metals and industrial chemicals, have also been linked to an increased risk of cancer.

But what we know goes beyond statistics and data. It's about understanding how pollution affects people's daily lives, how it infiltrates their homes, their workplaces, and even their children's play areas. It's about recognising that pollution and cancer are not just individual health problems, but also issues of social and environmental justice, disproportionately affecting poor and marginalised communities.

In short, what we know about cancer and pollution is a call to action. It is an invitation to rethink our relationship with our environment, to reassess our industrial practices and to adopt healthier, more sustainable lifestyles. It is a reminder that the fight against cancer is intrinsically linked to our fight for a cleaner and safer environment for all.

Purpose of the Book

The aim of this book, "Pollution and Cancer: A Toxic Relationship", is threefold: to inform, to raise awareness and to mobilise. It aims to provide a comprehensive and nuanced understanding of the link between pollution and cancer, highlighting the latest scientific research, real-life case studies and personal accounts. The book aims to be both an educational guide and a plea for collective action, highlighting the importance of prevention, regulation and societal responsibility in the fight against these two scourges.

Chapter 1

CANCER IN THE MODERN WORLD

Understanding Cancer: Definitions and Types

Cancer, often seen as a complex, multifactorial disease, is essentially characterised by the abnormal growth and proliferation of cells. To fully grasp the impact of pollution on cancer, it is crucial to first understand what cancer is, and its different types.

Definition of Cancer

Cancer is not a single disease, but a group of diseases linked by a common trait: the uncontrolled growth of abnormal cells. These cancer cells can invade adjacent tissues and spread to other parts of the body, a process known as metastasis. Unlike normal cells, cancer cells do not respond to the regulatory signals that control cell growth and division, leading to tumours and lesions in various organs.

Types of Cancer

Cancer comes in many forms, each affecting a different part of the body and having distinct characteristics:
- Cancers Carcinomas
    - These cancers develop in epithelial cells, which form the outer layer of the skin and certain internal tissues.
    - Common examples: breast cancer, lung cancer, prostate cancer and colorectal cancer.
- Sarcoma cancers
    - Sarcomas originate in supporting tissues such as bone, cartilage, fat, muscle and blood vessels.
    - Examples: osteosarcoma (bone) and liposarcoma (adipose tissue).
- Leukaemia
    - These cancers affect the tissues that form blood, such as bone marrow, and lead to the excessive production of abnormal blood cells.
    - Types: acute lymphocytic leukaemia, chronic myeloid leukaemia, etc.
- Lymphomas
    - Lymphomas affect the lymphatic system, a crucial part of the immune system.
    - Two main categories: Hodgkin's lymphoma and non-Hodgkin's lymphoma.
- Brain Cancers and Other Nervous System Tumours
    - These cancers affect the brain and spinal cord.

- Examples: glioma and astrocytoma.
- Melanoma and other skin cancers
    - These cancers develop from skin cells, in particular melanocytes, which are responsible for skin pigmentation.
- Cancers of the Reproductive Organs
    - Affects the reproductive organs, such as the ovaries and uterus in women, and the testicles and prostate gland in men.

Each type of cancer has its own characteristics, treatments and prognosis, making the fight against it all the more complex. Understanding these different types is fundamental to understanding how environmental factors, such as pollution, can influence their development and progression.

Cancer Risk Factors

The risk factors for cancer are many and varied, encompassing genetic, environmental, behavioural and even lifestyle factors. Understanding these factors is essential if we are to grasp the complexity of cancer and identify ways of preventing and reducing the risks.

Genetic factors

- **Heredity:** Certain types of cancer, such as breast, ovarian, colon and rectal, may run in families because of inherited genetic mutations.
- **Genetic predisposition:** Specific mutations in genes such as BRCA1 and BRCA2 increase the risk of certain cancers.

Environmental factors and exposure

- **Air pollution:** Fine particles and air pollutants are linked to an increased risk of lung cancer and other cancers.
- **Exposure to chemicals:** Substances such as asbestos, benzene, dioxins and certain pesticides have been classified as carcinogenic.
- **Radiation:** Exposure to ionising radiation (such as X-rays and gamma rays) and ultraviolet radiation can increase the risk of cancer.

Behavioural and lifestyle factors

- **Smoking:** Smoking is a major risk factor for lung cancer and also contributes to many other types of cancer.

- **Alcohol:** Excessive alcohol consumption is associated with an increased risk of cancers of the mouth, liver, breast, colon and rectum.
- **Diet and physical activity:** An unbalanced diet and lack of physical activity can increase the risk of certain types of cancer.
- **Obesity:** Obesity is a recognised risk factor for several types of cancer, including endometrial, breast, ovarian, colon and rectal cancer.

Infections

- **Viruses and bacteria:** Certain pathogens, such as the human papilloma virus (HPV), hepatitis B and C, and the Helicobacter pylori bacterium, are associated with an increased risk of cancer.

Age

- **Ageing:** The risk of developing cancer generally increases with age, due to the accumulation of genetic mutations over time and the reduced effectiveness of DNA repair mechanisms.

It is important to note that the presence of one or more of these risk factors does not mean that a person will necessarily develop cancer. Cancer is often the result of a complex interaction between numerous risk factors. In addition, many cancers develop in individuals with no known risk factors. However, knowledge and management of these factors can play a crucial role in the prevention and early detection of cancer.

The Evolution of Cancer Research

The evolution of cancer research is a fascinating story of discovery, innovation and continuous progress. It depicts a journey marked by major scientific advances, but also by challenges and lessons learned.

The beginnings of cancer research

- **Ancient origins:** The first mentions of cancer date back to Antiquity, but it was in the 19th century that scientific research into cancer really began.
- **Development of Cell Theory:** In the 19th century, the discovery that cancer arises from the transformation of normal cells laid the foundations for the modern understanding of cancer.

Advances in the 20th Century

- **Discovery of carcinogens:** The 20th century saw the identification of the first carcinogens, such as coal tar and tobacco.
- **Development of chemotherapy:** Chemotherapy was introduced in the middle of the 20th century, offering a new type of treatment for cancer.
- **Advances in radiology:** Improved radiography techniques have led to better diagnosis and treatment of cancer.

Genetics and Molecular Biology

- **Genetic revolution:** The end of the 20th century and the beginning of the 21st century have been marked by enormous progress in understanding the genetics of cancer.
- **Targeted therapies:** The advent of therapies specifically targeting genetic and molecular abnormalities in cancer cells has transformed the treatment of many types of cancer.

Immunotherapy and Advanced Treatments

- **Immunotherapy: In** recent years, immunotherapy, which uses the body's own immune system to fight cancer, has become a promising treatment option.
- **Personalised therapies:** Research is increasingly moving towards personalised treatments based on the specific genetic and molecular characteristics of tumours.

Current and future research

- **Multidisciplinary approaches:** Current cancer research involves a multidisciplinary approach, combining genetics, molecular biology, immunology and other fields.
- **Technology and Big Data:** The use of artificial intelligence and Big Data to analyse complex data sets is opening up new ways of understanding and treating cancer.
- **Prevention and screening:** There is also a growing emphasis on prevention, early screening and raising awareness of risk factors such as pollution.

The evolution of cancer research is an illustration of how science advances sometimes in leaps and bounds, sometimes incrementally, as researchers build on existing knowledge and explore new avenues. While many challenges remain, the story of cancer research is one of constant progress and renewed hope for the future.

Chapter 2

POLLUTION -
A
SILENT EVIL

What is Pollution?

Pollution, in its broadest sense, refers to the introduction into the environment of substances or factors that have a harmful effect on nature and living beings. It is a complex and multidimensional problem, affecting air, water, soil, and even noise and light. The impact of pollution is vast, ranging from the degradation of natural ecosystems to direct and serious effects on human health, including increased risk of diseases such as cancer.

Types of pollution

Air pollution :

From sources such as vehicle emissions, factories, power stations and even agricultural activities.

Includes pollutants such as fine particles (PM2.5 and PM10), sulphur dioxide, carbon monoxide and nitrogen oxides.

Water pollution :

Results from the discharge of harmful substances into rivers, lakes, oceans and groundwater.

This includes sewage, industrial waste, pesticides and herbicides from agriculture, and oil spills.

Soil pollution :

Occurs when chemicals or waste are spilt on the ground or buried.

Can come from agriculture (pesticides and fertilisers), industrial landfill sites and inadequate waste management.

Noise pollution :

Excessive noise from traffic, industrial activities, buildings and even leisure activities.

Can cause stress, sleep disturbances and other health problems.

Light pollution :

Excessive artificial lighting, particularly in urban areas.

Impacts the natural cycles of animals and can have effects on human health.

Thermal pollution :

Abnormal rise in temperature in the environment, often due to industrial processes.

Affects aquatic ecosystems and can alter the life cycles of species.

Radioactive pollution :

    The release of radioactive substances into the environment, often in connection with nuclear energy or nuclear accidents.

    Has long-term effects on health and the environment.

Causes and Consequences

Pollution is mainly caused by human activities, although natural sources such as volcanic eruptions also contribute. Its consequences are diverse: degradation of natural habitats, loss of biodiversity, climate change, and effects on human health such as respiratory diseases, heart disease and cancer.

In the context of this book, pollution is examined specifically for its role in increasing the risk of cancer, underlining the importance of understanding and controlling sources of pollution to protect public health and the environment.

The main sources of pollution

The main sources of pollution are diverse and extend across multiple sectors of human activity. Understanding these sources is crucial if we are to tackle pollution prevention and reduction effectively. Here is an overview of the major sources of pollution:

Industry:

    Industrial emissions: Factories and production facilities often release pollutants into the air, water and soil, including heavy metals, toxic chemicals and fine particles.

    Industrial waste: Inadequate management of industrial waste can lead to the contamination of vast areas, affecting ecosystems and human health.

Transport :

    Motor vehicles: Cars, lorries, motorbikes, planes and boats emit exhaust gases containing harmful substances such as nitrogen oxides, carbon monoxide and hydrocarbons.

Transport infrastructure: The construction and maintenance of roads, airports and seaports can also contribute to environmental pollution.

Agriculture :

Pesticides and herbicides: The intensive use of chemicals in agriculture can contaminate water, soil and food products.

Livestock: Livestock farms produce significant quantities of organic waste, which can pollute waterways and release greenhouse gases.

Energy :

Power stations: Power stations that run on coal, natural gas or oil are major sources of carbon dioxide emissions and other atmospheric pollutants.

Resource extraction and processing: The extraction of oil, natural gas and minerals can lead to spills, leaks and other forms of contamination.

Deforestation and urbanisation :

Deforestation: The removal of vast tracts of forest for agriculture, housing or industry reduces nature's ability to filter pollutants.

Urban expansion: Growing urbanisation is leading to an increase in pollution from construction, traffic and other urban activities.

Household and industrial waste :

Waste management: Landfill sites, waste incineration and inappropriate disposal of household chemicals contribute to soil and water pollution.

Mining activities :

Mining: The extraction of minerals and metals can lead to the contamination of water and soil by toxic substances.

Digital pollution :

Information technology: Data centres, massive use of the Internet and electronic equipment consume large quantities of energy and generate heat.

These sources of pollution often interact, creating complex environmental problems that require integrated solutions. Awareness of these sources and their effective management are essential to reduce environmental impact and protect public health.

Effects of Pollution on Human Health

Pollution has a profound and often devastating impact on human health, affecting almost every aspect of physical and mental well-being. The effects of pollution vary according to the nature and intensity of exposure to pollutants, as well as individual characteristics such as age, state of health and genetics. Here is an overview of the main effects of pollution on human health:

Respiratory effects

Respiratory diseases: Air pollution, particularly fine particles and gaseous pollutants, can cause or exacerbate respiratory diseases such as asthma, chronic bronchitis and chronic obstructive pulmonary disease (COPD).

Lung cancer: Prolonged exposure to certain pollutants, such as fine particles and carcinogenic compounds in the air, significantly increases the risk of lung cancer.

Cardiovascular effects

Heart disease: Pollution can contribute to cardiovascular problems, including coronary heart disease, heart attacks and strokes.

Hypertension: Chronic exposure to air pollution has been associated with an increase in blood pressure and an increased risk of hypertension.

Effects on Reproductive Health

Fertility problems: Certain pollutants, such as heavy metals and endocrine disruptors, can affect fertility in both men and women.

Effects on foetal development: Exposure to pollution during pregnancy can lead to complications such as premature birth, low birth weight and congenital anomalies.

Neurological effects

Neurological disorders: Studies suggest a link between pollution and neurological disorders such as Alzheimer's disease, Parkinson's disease and cognitive impairment.

Brain development in children: Early exposure to certain pollutants can affect children's brain development, leading to developmental delays and learning disabilities.

Dermatological effects

Skin problems: Pollution can cause or aggravate skin problems such as eczema, psoriasis and acne.

Psychological effects

Stress and anxiety: Noise and air pollution can increase stress and anxiety, affecting mental well-being.

Depression: Studies have found associations between pollution and an increased prevalence of depressive symptoms.

Other effects

Immune system: Pollution can weaken the immune system, making people more susceptible to infection.

Longevity and Quality of Life: Continued exposure to pollution can reduce life expectancy and lower overall quality of life.

These effects underline the importance of pollution control in protecting public health. Reducing pollution is not only an environmental issue, but also an urgent necessity to improve the health and well-being of people around the world.

Chapter 3

LINKING POLLUTION AND CANCER

Scientific Evidence of the Link

The existence of a link between pollution and cancer is solidly supported by a growing body of scientific evidence. This evidence comes from various epidemiological studies, clinical research and toxicological analyses. Here are some key aspects of this evidence:

Epidemiological studies

Correlation between Pollution and Cancer Incidence: Numerous epidemiological studies have shown a correlation between exposure to pollution and an increased incidence of certain types of cancer, in particular lung, bladder and breast cancer.

Cohort and case-control studies: These studies follow large groups of people over long periods or compare individuals exposed to pollutants with unexposed individuals, providing evidence of the link between exposure to pollution and cancer risk.

Clinical and Toxicological Research

Carcinogenic effects of pollutants : Clinical and toxicological research has identified several substances present in pollution (such as benzene, asbestos and certain aromatic polycyclic hydrocarbons) as carcinogenic.

Biological mechanisms: Studies have shown how these substances can damage DNA, cause mutations and disrupt the normal functioning of cells, leading to the development of cancer.

Reports and Assessments of Healthcare Organisations

WHO and IARC classification of pollutants: The World Health Organisation (WHO) and the International Agency for Research on Cancer (IARC) have classified several pollutants as carcinogenic to humans, based on scientific evidence.

Global assessments: These organisations also provide global assessments of the risks associated with pollution, reinforcing the link between pollution and cancer.

Case Studies and Anecdotal Reports

High pollution areas: Case studies in areas with high industrial or urban pollution often show higher than average cancer rates.

Testimonies from Affected Communities : Although anecdotal, the testimonies of people living in polluted areas offer human perspectives that corroborate the scientific data.

Advances in biomarkers and imaging

Early detection: The development of biomarkers and advanced imaging techniques has led to a better understanding and early detection of the carcinogenic effects of pollution.

This evidence forms a solid basis for affirming that pollution is a significant risk factor for cancer. It underlines the importance of policies and practices aimed at reducing pollution in order to protect public health.

Biological and chemical mechanisms

The biological and chemical mechanisms by which pollution contributes to the development of cancer are complex and involve several pathways at cellular and molecular level. Here is an overview of these mechanisms:

Genotoxicity and DNA mutations

DNA damage: Many pollutants are genotoxic, which means that they can directly damage the DNA of cells. This alteration can cause genetic mutations that lead to cancerous cell transformation.

Free radicals: Certain pollutants, such as fine particles, can generate free radicals that damage DNA, proteins and cellular lipids, thereby contributing to carcinogenesis.

Endocrine disruption

Endocrine disrupters: Some pollutants act as endocrine disruptors, mimicking or interfering with the body's natural hormones. This can unbalance the hormonal processes regulating cell growth and reproduction, increasing the risk of hormone-dependent cancers such as breast and prostate cancer.

Chronic inflammation

Inflammatory response: Exposure to certain pollutants can cause chronic inflammation, which, if it persists, can encourage the growth and spread of cancer cells.

Cytokines and growth factors: Chronic inflammation can lead to an increase in cytokines and growth factors, which can stimulate cell division and inhibit the processes of programmed cell death (apoptosis), thereby promoting cancer.

Immunosuppression
> **Weakening of the immune system:** Certain pollutants can weaken the immune system, reducing its ability to detect and destroy cancer cells or repair DNA damage.

Activation of Oncogenes and Inactivation of Tumour Suppressor Genes
> **Genetic changes:** Pollution can lead to the activation of oncogenes (genes which, when mutated or expressed at abnormal levels, can lead to cancer) and the inactivation of tumour suppressor genes, thus disrupting the normal control of cell growth.

Impaired Cellular Communication
> **Cell signalling:** Pollutants can disrupt the cell signalling pathways that regulate cell growth, division and death, leading to uncontrolled cell proliferation.

Epigenetics
> **Epigenetic modifications:** Some pollutants can induce epigenetic modifications (changes in gene expression without altering the DNA sequence), thus influencing cell behaviour in a way that may be conducive to the development of cancer.

These mechanisms show how environmental pollutants can initiate or promote the carcinogenic process at various levels of cellular and molecular biology. Understanding these mechanisms is essential for developing effective strategies for preventing and treating pollution-related cancer.

Case study: Highly polluted areas

Highly polluted areas provide crucial case studies for understanding the impact of pollution on human health, particularly in terms of increased risk of cancer. These case studies often highlight striking correlations between high levels of pollution and a high incidence of certain diseases, including various types of cancer. Here are some notable examples:

1. Ruhr Industrial Valley in Germany
> **History:** One of the most densely populated industrial areas in Europe, known for its steelworks and coal mines.

Health problems: Studies have shown high rates of respiratory disease and cancer, particularly lung cancer, linked to air pollution and industrial emissions.

2. Triangle of Death in Italy

Location: This region around Naples is infamous for its high incidence of cancer, attributed to the illegal management of industrial waste and water and soil pollution.

Findings: Research has revealed a link between exposure to toxic substances in the environment and an increased risk of several types of cancer.

3. Bhopal, India

Disaster: The 1984 disaster at the Union Carbide plant released toxic gas, causing immediate deaths and long-term health problems.

Consequences: The survivors and their descendants suffered from various health problems, including a higher rate of cancer, attributed to prolonged exposure to the toxins.

4. Appalachian Basin in the United States

Context: The region is known for its intensive coal mining, which generates air and water pollution.

Impact on health: High rates of lung cancer and other respiratory diseases have been documented, often linked to air quality and exposure to fine particles.

5. Chernobyl, Ukraine

Nuclear accident: The 1986 disaster resulted in the release of radioactive materials into the environment.

Health effects: Increase in cases of thyroid cancer, particularly in children, due to exposure to radiation.

6. Niger Delta

Oil pollution: This oil extraction region suffers from water and soil pollution due to oil spills.

Health consequences: Local communities have high rates of various health problems, including cancer, potentially linked to pollution.

These case studies show that people living in highly polluted areas often face an increased risk of developing cancer and other serious illnesses. They underline the importance of environmental monitoring, strict pollution regulations and the implementation of decontamination measures to protect public health.

Chapter 4

TESTIMONIES AND REALITIES

Life Stories: Victims of Pollution

The life stories of pollution victims tell often poignant tales, highlighting the direct human impacts of environmental contamination. These personal accounts provide an essential perspective on the real consequences of pollution, going far beyond statistics and clinical studies. Here are a few illustrative examples:

1. Farmers affected by pesticides

Context: In many agricultural regions, the intensive use of pesticides has led to water and soil contamination.

Testimonial: A farmer develops a rare form of cancer after years of exposure to pesticides. He describes how he had to battle not only the disease, but also isolation and the challenge of making his community aware of the dangers of the chemicals they use every day.

2. Residents of Industrial Zones

Situation: People living near large industrial plants are often exposed to highly polluted air.

Story: A family living near a steelworks shares their experience with several family members suffering from chronic respiratory problems and cancer. They express their feelings of powerlessness in the face of a deteriorating environmental situation and the lack of satisfactory responses from the authorities.

3. Survivors of Environmental Disasters

Event: Disasters such as oil spills or major industrial accidents have long-term health consequences.

Story: A survivor of such a disaster talks about the immediate impact on his health and that of his community, including chronic illness and cancer, as well as continuing economic and psychological difficulties.

4. Children and Families in Polluted Cities

Setting: Urban areas with high levels of air pollution present particular risks for children.

Experience: Parents describe their daily struggle to protect the health of their asthmatic child in a city with dangerously high pollution levels, highlighting the difficulty of making lifestyle choices when faced with economic and social constraints.

5. Indigenous populations and contaminated resources

Context: Indigenous communities are often affected by the pollution of the natural resources on which they depend.

Story: A member of an indigenous community shares how contamination of water and land by mining activities has not only caused health problems such as cancer, but has also eroded their traditional way of life and culture.

These individual stories highlight the human dimension of pollution - the challenges, struggles and losses experienced by individuals and communities. They are a poignant reminder that behind every statistic on pollution and cancer, there are real people, with their own stories, hopes and fears.

Fighting Communities

Communities fighting pollution and its health consequences, such as cancer, represent stories of resilience, solidarity and sometimes success in the face of considerable environmental challenges. These communities, often located near sources of industrial pollution or in neglected areas, are mobilising to defend their right to a healthy environment. Here are a few examples of their struggles:

1. Collective action against industrial pollution

Situation: Communities located near factories or industrial complexes suffer from high levels of air or water pollution.

Fighting: These communities organise demonstrations, petitions and legal action to demand reductions in polluting emissions and better environmental regulation. They often work with NGOs and experts to document health impacts and strengthen their cases.

2. Cleaning and Environmental Restoration

Context: Areas contaminated by decades of industrial and mining activity.

Mobilisation: Residents join forces to demand the clean-up and rehabilitation of their environment. These efforts can include raising funds for independent environmental studies and pressuring governments to intervene.

3. Health Promotion and Cancer Prevention

Challenge: In areas of high pollution, cancer rates can be high.

Action: Communities set up cancer awareness programmes, free screening and health promotion initiatives to encourage preventive behaviour and facilitate early diagnosis.

4. Resistance to Polluting Projects

Issue: Proposals for new industrial or expansion projects that threaten to increase pollution.

Answer: Communities are organising themselves to resist these projects through information campaigns, demonstrations and legal action, often highlighting the risks to public health.

5. Environmental education and awareness

Need: A lack of awareness and education about the impacts of pollution.

Initiatives: Educational programmes are being launched to inform residents about the risks of pollution, ways of reducing exposure and the importance of environmental monitoring.

6. Collaboration with scientists and experts

Strategy: To strengthen their cause, communities often collaborate with researchers and public health experts.

Result: These collaborations make it possible to carry out epidemiological and environmental studies that provide the scientific evidence needed to back up their claims and actions.

These community struggles demonstrate the ability of people affected by pollution to organise and demand meaningful change. They also illustrate the importance of civic engagement, community solidarity and mutual support in managing environmental and health challenges.

Psychological and social repercussions

The psychological and social repercussions of pollution, particularly when associated with increased risks of serious illnesses such as cancer, are profound and often underestimated. These impacts go beyond the immediate physical consequences, affecting the quality of life, mental well-being and social cohesion of individuals and communities. Some of these impacts include

Stress and Anxiety

Constant anxiety: Living in polluted areas can lead to chronic anxiety about personal health and that of loved ones, especially when there is a high risk of diseases such as cancer.

Fear of the future: Fear of the long-term consequences of exposure to pollution, both for health and the environment, can be a constant source of stress.

Effects on Mental Health

Depression: Awareness of health risks and environmental degradation can lead to feelings of despair and depression, particularly among those who feel powerless to change their situation.

Trauma: People affected by pollution-related environmental disasters can suffer lasting psychological trauma.

Impact on Community Cohesion

Conflicts and tensions: Pollution can be a source of conflict within communities, particularly when there are disagreements about causes, responsibilities and measures to be taken.

Sense of abandonment: Communities that feel neglected or abandoned by the authorities or companies responsible for pollution may feel isolated and distrustful.

Effects on children and families

Child development: Children living in polluted environments can be particularly vulnerable to psychological effects, affecting their emotional and social development.

Family dynamics: The illness of a family member due to pollution can change roles and dynamics within the family, sometimes leading to additional financial and emotional pressures.

Economic and social consequences

Loss of Income and Employment: Pollution can affect livelihoods, particularly in resource-dependent communities, increasing economic stress.

Marginalisation and Environmental Injustice: Poor and marginalised communities are often the hardest hit by pollution, exacerbating social and economic inequalities.

Effects on Quality of Life
> **Daily restrictions:** Pollution can limit outdoor activities, social interaction and access to healthy environments, reducing overall quality of life.

These repercussions show that the effects of pollution extend far beyond physical health, profoundly affecting the social and psychological fabric of individuals and communities. Taking these aspects into account is essential for a comprehensive and effective response to pollution and its consequences.

Chapter 5

THE SCIENCE BEHIND THE FACTS

Recent Research and Discoveries

Recent research into pollution and its link with cancer has led to a number of important discoveries. These advances are improving our understanding of how pollution affects human health and paving the way for new prevention and treatment strategies. Here are some of the most relevant discoveries and research:

Advances in Understanding Molecular Mechanisms

Cellular interactions: Recent studies have highlighted the complex interactions between pollutants and human cells, including how certain pollutants modify DNA or disrupt cellular processes.

Biomarkers of exposure: The development of biomarkers to measure exposure to certain pollutants is helping to establish a more direct link between exposure to pollution and the risk of cancer.

Air Pollution and Cancer Risks

Ultrafine particles: Research has deepened our understanding of the health effects of ultrafine particles (less than 2.5 micrometres), showing a clearer link with specific cancers, notably lung cancer.

Indoor pollution: Increased attention is being paid to indoor air pollution, including the risks associated with second-hand smoke, heating and cooking appliances, and building materials.

Impact of Emerging Pollutants

Microplastics: Studying the impact of microplastics, particularly their presence in food chains and their potential carcinogenic effect, has become an important area of research.

New Chemical Pollutants: Research is extending to lesser-known or emerging pollutants, such as flame retardants, specific industrial chemicals and nanoparticles.

Detection and Purification Technologies

Environmental monitoring: The development of advanced technologies for monitoring air and water pollution is helping to identify and quantify the risks to human health.

Air and water purification: Advances in purification and filtration methods offer new ways of reducing exposure to pollutants.

Effects of Pollution on Overall Health
> **Large-scale studies:** Large-scale research projects, such as those incorporating public health and environmental data, provide valuable information on the long-term effects of pollution on various populations.

Preventive and regulatory approaches
> **Public health policies:** Research informs public health policies aimed at reducing pollution and protecting vulnerable populations.
>
> **Prevention and awareness:** Educational and prevention programmes based on recent scientific data are increasingly being adopted to raise public awareness of the risks associated with pollution.

These discoveries and research underline the dynamic and constantly evolving nature of the field of pollution and human health. They offer new perspectives for tackling the challenges posed by pollution and open up promising avenues for the prevention and treatment of pollution-related diseases, including cancer.

Pollutants and Specific Carcinogens

Understanding pollutants and specific carcinogens is essential for assessing and managing the risks associated with pollution. Many pollutants have been identified as carcinogens, meaning that they have the capacity to cause or promote the development of cancer. Here are some of the most notorious pollutants and carcinogens:

Air Pollutants
> **Fine particles (PM2.5 and PM10):** Suspended in the air, these particles can penetrate deep into the lungs and even enter the bloodstream, increasing the risk of lung cancer.
>
> **Benzene:** Found in tobacco smoke, petrol and industrial emissions, benzene is a known carcinogen, linked to blood cancers such as leukaemia.
>
> **Asbestos :** Exposure to asbestos, mainly in the workplace, is a well-established cause of mesothelioma (a cancer of the pleura) and lung cancer.

Water Pollutants

Arsenic: Present in certain sources of drinking water, arsenic can cause skin, bladder and lung cancer.

Nitrates: Used in agricultural fertilisers, they can end up in drinking water and have been linked to an increased risk of certain types of cancer, particularly stomach cancer.

Soil Pollutants and Food Contaminants

Dioxins and PCBs (Polychlorinated biphenyls): These environmental contaminants can accumulate in the food chain and are linked to several types of cancer.

Pesticides and herbicides: Certain chemicals used in agriculture, such as glyphosate, have been controversial for their potential links with cancer.

Industrial Chemicals

Polycyclic Aromatic Hydrocarbons (PAHs): Present in smoke, tar and certain industrial products, PAHs are known carcinogens.

Heavy metals: Lead, cadmium and mercury, often present in contaminated industrial sites, can increase the risk of certain cancers.

Indoor Pollutants

Radon: This naturally occurring radioactive gas, which can accumulate in houses, is the second leading cause of lung cancer after smoking.

Tobacco smoke: Second-hand smoke is a mixture of more than 7,000 chemical substances, several of which are carcinogenic.

Occupational Risk Factors

Specific Occupational Exposures: Certain occupations, particularly in the chemical, steel and construction industries, expose workers to increased risks of cancer due to exposure to specific substances.

Recognition and regulation of these pollutants and carcinogens are crucial to cancer prevention. Efforts to reduce exposure to these substances, whether through personal protection measures, changes to industrial processes, or government regulations, are essential to improving public health.

Scientific challenges and prospects

Research into the relationship between pollution and cancer, although progressing rapidly, is faced with a number of scientific challenges and perspectives. These challenges need to be addressed if we are to gain a deeper understanding and develop effective prevention and treatment strategies. Here are some of the main challenges and opportunities in this field:

Scientific Challenges
  Exhibition complexity :
        Pollution comes in many forms (air, water, soil) and individuals are often exposed to a mixture of pollutants, which makes it difficult to understand the specific effects on health.
  Causal links :
        Establishing a direct causal link between exposure to specific pollutants and the development of cancer is difficult, due to the long latency of cancer and the influence of other risk factors.

  Individual variability :
        Genetic differences between individuals can affect the way they react to pollution, making it difficult to generalise the results.
  Exposure Metering :
        Accurately   measuring long-term exposure to low levels of pollutants remains a challenge, requiring advanced technologies and methodologies.
Outlook
  Surveillance and Detection   Technologies :
        The development of more sensitive technologies for monitoring and detecting environmental pollutants will provide more accurate data for research.
  Integrated and Multidisciplinary   Approaches :
        Integrated   approaches combining epidemiology, toxicology, molecular biology and genetics can lead to a better understanding of the mechanisms by which pollution influences cancer.

Prevention and awareness :
> Improving public awareness and developing prevention strategies based on current scientific evidence can help reduce the burden of pollution-related cancer.

Data-driven   policies :
> Research data can inform public policy and regulations aimed at controlling and reducing pollution.

Global collaboration :
> Pollution and cancer are global problems. International collaboration on research and data sharing can lead to significant advances.

Innovations in Treatment :
> Research could also focus on developing more effective treatments for cancers specifically linked to pollution.

By overcoming these challenges and exploiting these opportunities, science can move towards a better understanding and management of the impact of pollution on cancer, leading to significant improvements in the prevention, diagnosis and treatment of this complex and multifaceted disease.

Chapter 6

PREVENTION AND ACTION

Prevention and safety measures

Prevention and safety measures are essential to reduce the risks of cancer associated with pollution. These measures involve a combination of actions at different levels - individual, community and governmental. Here are some key strategies:

Individual level
    Reducing Personal Exposure:
        Avoid areas of high atmospheric pollution, especially during strenuous exercise.
        Use air purifiers in the home, especially in polluted urban areas.
    Healthy Lifestyle Choices :
        Eat a diet rich in fruit and vegetables, and low in processed foods and red meat.
        Stop smoking and avoid second-hand smoke.
    Awareness-raising and education :
        Keep informed about local pollution risks and ways of reducing exposure.
        Participate in health awareness and cancer screening programmes.
At Community level
    Air and water quality   monitoring :
        Set up local monitoring systems to inform residents of pollution levels.
        Encourage community participation in monitoring and reporting pollution problems.
    Collective actions :
        Organise clean-up campaigns and tree planting to improve the quality of the local environment.
        Engage in advocacy for better environmental regulation.
At government and institutional level
    Regulations and standards :
        Impose strict standards for industrial emissions, motor vehicles and hazardous chemicals.
        Strengthen laws and controls on the management of industrial and household waste.
    Promoting Clean Energy and Sustainable Technologies:
        Encouraging the use of renewable energies and less polluting technologies.
        Subsidise research and development into pollution-reduction technologies.

Public Health   Programmes :
> Implement national campaigns to raise awareness of the risks associated with pollution.
> Offer accessible cancer screening and prevention programmes.

International partnerships :
> Working with other countries and international organisations to address transboundary pollution issues.

These measures, when implemented in a consistent and sustained manner, can play a significant role in reducing exposure to pollution and, consequently, in reducing the risk of cancer. They require the commitment and collaboration of all sectors of society.

Public Health Policy and Role of Government

Public health policies and the role of governments are fundamental in the fight against pollution and the prevention of cancer associated with it. Government authorities can play a number of key roles, from regulating and controlling pollution to raising awareness and supporting research. Here are some key aspects of these policies and roles:

Regulation and Control
> **Air and Water Quality Standards:** Setting and enforcing strict standards to limit the levels of pollutants in the air and water.
> **Regulation of Industrial Emissions:** Imposing limits on emissions from factories, power stations and other industrial sources.
> **Waste management: Implement** effective policies for the management and treatment of industrial and household waste, including toxic substances.

Awareness-raising and education
> **Information campaigns:** Launch public awareness campaigns on the health risks of pollution and ways of reducing personal exposure.
> **Educational programmes:** Integrate environmental education into school curricula to raise awareness from an early age.

Support for Research and Development
Research funding: Allocate funds for research into the effects of pollution on health and into new technologies for monitoring and reducing pollution.
Scientific collaboration: Encouraging collaboration between universities, research institutes and the private sector to promote innovation in the field of environmental health.
Public Health Policy
Cancer screening programmes: Setting up and promoting early detection programmes for pollution-related cancers.
Preventive Health Interventions: Developing public health initiatives focused on cancer prevention, including recommendations on lifestyle and diet.
International collaboration
Environmental agreements: Participating in international agreements and initiatives to combat pollution on a global scale.
Exchange of best practice: sharing knowledge and experience of pollution regulation and control with other countries.
Local and regional actions
Urban policies: Promoting sustainable urban policies, such as improving public transport and creating low-emission zones.
Community support: Working directly with local communities to identify and resolve specific pollution problems.

By adopting a holistic and multi-dimensional approach, governments can play a decisive role in reducing exposure to pollution and, consequently, in reducing the risk of cancer. These efforts require close cooperation between different government sectors, the private sector, communities and international organisations.

Community mobilisation and awareness-raising

Community mobilisation and awareness-raising are crucial in the fight against pollution and cancer prevention. These efforts involve the active engagement of local communities to identify, understand and act on the pollution problems that affect them. Here are some key strategies:

Education and awareness
Workshops and Seminars: Organising educational events to inform residents about the risks of pollution and how to protect themselves.
Educational resources: Distribute brochures, posters and online resources to raise awareness of the effects of pollution on health.
Awareness campaigns
Media campaigns: Use local media, social networks and other platforms to disseminate information about pollution and cancer.
Awareness days: Organise theme days focusing on environmental health to raise public awareness.

Participation and Community Involvement
Working groups: Set up working groups or committees to tackle specific pollution problems in the community.
Public Forums: Hold meetings where residents can discuss environmental concerns and propose solutions.
Working with Local Authorities
Advocacy: Working with local authorities to develop policies and regulations to reduce pollution.
Partnerships: Establish partnerships with schools, hospitals and local businesses for joint pollution reduction initiatives.
Environmental Monitoring Initiatives
Citizen Monitoring Programmes: Encouraging residents to take part in monitoring air and water quality.
Applications and technologies: Using mobile applications and other technologies to enable citizens to report pollution problems.
Collective actions
Demonstrations and petitions: Organise peaceful demonstrations and petitions to draw attention to specific pollution problems.
Clean-up and Reforestation: Carrying out clean-up campaigns and tree-planting projects to improve the local environment.

Community Capacity Building

Training and Resources: Providing training and resources to help communities manage pollution problems effectively.

Support networks: Build support networks to share experience, knowledge and resources between affected communities.

Community mobilisation and awareness-raising play a vital role in creating a healthier environment and preventing pollution-related diseases such as cancer. When communities are informed and engaged, they can become powerful agents of change and advocates for a better quality of life.

Chapter 7

ENVIRONMENTAL IMPACT AND CANCER

Climate Change and Pollution

Climate change and pollution are closely linked, each influencing and exacerbating the other. This interaction poses unique challenges for both the environment and human health. Here are some key aspects of the relationship between climate change and pollution:

Exacerbated Effects of Climate Change on Pollution

Air quality: Higher temperatures due to climate change can increase ground-level ozone, a dangerous air pollutant that exacerbates respiratory and cardiovascular problems.

Pollutant Spread: Extreme weather conditions, such as storms and floods, can spread pollutants over greater distances, increasing exposure in previously less affected areas.

Impact of Pollution on Climate Change

Greenhouse gases: Atmospheric pollutants, particularly carbon dioxide (CO_2) and methane (CH_4), are major greenhouse gases that contribute to global warming.

Albedo and warming: Some pollutants, such as soot particles, can affect the Earth's albedo (reflection of sunlight), influencing the climate.

Combined Effects on Human Health

Increase in disease: The combination of pollution and climate change can lead to an increase in respiratory illnesses, heat stroke, heart disease and cancer.

Food Security and Water: Climate change is affecting the availability and quality of water and food, which can have an impact on human health, particularly in vulnerable regions.

Challenges for Ecosystems

Biodiversity loss: Climate change and pollution can degrade natural habitats, threatening biodiversity and essential ecosystem services.

Ocean pollution: Ocean acidification due to CO_2 absorption, combined with pollution from plastics and chemicals, is having a serious impact on marine life.

Socio-economic issues

Inequalities: The effects of climate change and pollution are not evenly distributed, hitting poor and vulnerable communities hardest.

Climate migration: The combined impacts on the environment and health can force populations to migrate, creating climate refugees.

Integrated Solutions

Environmental policies: Integrated policies that address both pollution and climate change are necessary for effective management.

Green Technologies: The development and adoption of clean and renewable technologies can reduce polluting emissions while mitigating climate change.

In summary, the relationship between climate change and pollution is a complex cycle where each problem reinforces the other. Understanding and concerted action on both fronts are essential to protect both the environment and public health.

Effects of environmental disasters on Health

Environmental disasters, whether caused by human activities or natural phenomena, have profound and often lasting effects on human health. These effects can be direct and immediate, but also indirect and long-term. Here is an overview of the health consequences of these disasters:

Direct and Immediate Effects

Injuries and deaths: Industrial accidents, chemical spills, earthquakes, floods and hurricanes can cause immediate physical injury and sometimes death.

Respiratory problems: Forest fires, volcanic eruptions and chemical accidents can release toxic particles and gases into the air, causing acute respiratory problems.

Indirect and long-term effects

Chronic diseases: Prolonged exposure to pollutants released during disasters can increase the risk of chronic diseases, including cancer, respiratory and cardiovascular diseases.

Psychological problems: Disasters can cause significant stress and anxiety, leading to psychological disorders such as post-traumatic stress disorder (PTSD), depression and anxiety.

Impact on healthcare systems

Overload of health services: Environmental disasters can overload local health systems, hindering access to necessary medical care and treatment.

Loss of infrastructure: The destruction of health infrastructure can limit access to healthcare, drinking water and sanitation, exacerbating public health problems.

Risks of epidemics and infectious diseases

Spread of disease: Post-disaster conditions such as stagnant water and population displacement can encourage the spread of infectious diseases such as cholera, dengue fever and malaria.

Vaccination disruption: Disasters can interrupt vaccination programmes, increasing the risk of outbreaks of vaccine-preventable diseases.

Effects on Mental Health

Emotional trauma: The loss of loved ones, homes and livelihoods can have a devastating impact on people's mental health.

Impact on Communities: Affected communities may experience a sense of loss and despair, affecting social cohesion and mutual support.

Consequences for nutrition and diet

Food insecurity: Disruptions to food production and distribution can lead to malnutrition, particularly among children and vulnerable populations.

Drinking water: Contamination of drinking water can cause gastrointestinal illness and other health problems.

Effects on Vulnerable Populations

Children and the elderly: These groups are particularly vulnerable to the effects of disasters, both physically and psychologically.

Low Income Communities: Poor communities are often the hardest hit, as they have fewer resources to prepare for, respond to and recover from disasters.

By recognising and understanding these various effects, governments, humanitarian organisations and communities can better prepare for and respond to environmental disasters, thereby minimising their negative impact on human health.

Biodiversity, Ecosystems and Their Links with Cancer

Biodiversity and the health of ecosystems play a crucial role in human health, including the prevention and control of cancer. The destruction of ecosystems and the loss of biodiversity can have direct and indirect repercussions on the incidence of cancer. Here are some aspects of this relationship:

The Role of Ecosystems in Pollutant Regulation

Natural filtration: Ecosystems such as forests, wetlands and oceans act as natural filters, absorbing and breaking down pollutants that may be carcinogenic to humans.

Reducing Air Pollution: Plants and trees absorb harmful air pollutants, helping to improve air quality and reduce the risk of respiratory cancers.

Loss of Biodiversity and Health Risks

Ecological imbalances: The loss of biodiversity can lead to ecological imbalances that encourage the proliferation of certain disease-carrying species or the concentration of pollutants.

Loss of Natural Sources of Medicines : Many drugs, including those used in chemotherapy, are derived from compounds found in nature. The loss of biodiversity reduces the potential for discovering new cancer treatments.

Interactions between Climate Change, Ecosystems and Cancer

Modification of disease distribution areas: Climate change, by altering ecosystems, can extend the distribution areas of certain infectious diseases, which are sometimes risk factors for certain types of cancer.

Environmental stress: Changes in ecosystems due to climate change can increase the concentration of certain pollutants or alter their distribution, thus indirectly affecting the risk of cancer.

Ecosystem Services and Cancer Prevention

Food and Nutrition: Healthy ecosystems provide a diversity of foods rich in nutrients and phytochemicals essential for cancer prevention.

Mental and physical well-being: Access to healthy natural environments encourages physical activity and mental well-being, two important factors in cancer prevention.

Research and Education
> **Epidemiological studies:** Research is needed to better understand how ecosystem health affects the incidence of cancer in humans.

> **Raising awareness:** Educating the public about the importance of conserving biodiversity and ecosystems for human health, including cancer prevention.

Preserving and restoring ecosystems and biodiversity is essential not only for the environment, but also for human health. By recognising and acting on these links, we can help both to protect our planet and to fight cancer.

Chapter 8

INVISIBLE POLLUTION

Sound and Light Pollution and Their Effects

Noise and light pollution, although often less visible than other forms of pollution, have significant effects on human health and the environment. Here is an overview of their impact:

Sound pollution
> Effects on Hearing Health :
>> **Hearing loss:** Prolonged exposure to high levels of noise can lead to permanent hearing loss.
>> **Tinnitus:** Constant or loud noises can cause ringing or whistling in the ears.
>
> Effects on General Health :
>> **Stress and heart disease:** Excessive noise can increase stress, blood pressure and the risk of heart disease.
>> **Sleep disturbance:** Noise at night can disrupt sleep, leading to fatigue, irritability and concentration problems.
>
> Psychological effects :
>> **Anxiety and depression:** High noise levels can increase the risk of mental disorders such as anxiety and depression.

Light pollution
> Effects on Circadian Rhythms:
>> **Sleep disruption:** Artificial light, particularly blue light from screens, can disrupt circadian rhythms and affect sleep quality.
>> **Health Consequences:** Disruption of circadian rhythms can be linked to a variety of health problems, including obesity, diabetes and even certain types of cancer, such as breast cancer.
>
> Impact on wildlife :
>> **Animal orientation:** Artificial light can disorientate nocturnal animals, migratory birds and insects, affecting their breeding and migration habits.
>> **Disrupted ecosystems:** Light pollution can disrupt ecosystems by affecting food chains and natural behaviour.

Consequences for Mental Health :

Reduced well-being: Reduced visibility of the stars and night sky can affect psychological well-being and connection with nature.

Managing Sound and Light Pollution

Reducing noise sources: Using sound-absorbing materials in construction, limiting noise from vehicles and industrial activities, and establishing quiet zones in urban areas.

Lighting control: Use limited, directed outdoor lighting to reduce light pollution, encourage the use of light sources that are less disruptive to circadian rhythms, and turn off unnecessary lights at night.

Awareness and management of noise and light pollution are essential to protect human health and preserve natural environments. Policies and practices aimed at reducing these forms of pollution can significantly improve quality of life and contribute to a healthier environment.

Microscopic pollutants and nanoparticles

Microscopic pollutants, particularly nanoparticles, have become a growing concern because of their ability to penetrate deep into human and environmental biological systems. Here is an overview of their characteristics and effects:

Nature and sources of nanoparticles

Size and composition: Nanoparticles are extremely small, generally measuring between 1 and 100 nanometres. They can be composed of various materials, such as metals, carbon or chemical compounds.

Industrial sources: These are often produced by industrial processes, the combustion of fossil fuels, vehicle exhausts and certain manufacturing processes.

Nanotechnologies: The growing use of nanotechnologies in various fields (medicine, electronics, materials) has also increased the presence of nanoparticles in the environment.

Penetration and accumulation in the body

Deep penetration: Because of their tiny size, nanoparticles can penetrate deep into the lungs, crossing cell barriers and even reaching the bloodstream.

Bioaccumulation: There is a risk of bioaccumulation in tissues, which could lead to long-term toxic effects.

Health effects

Respiratory and cardiovascular problems: Inhalation of nanoparticles can cause acute and chronic respiratory problems and contribute to cardiovascular disease.

Carcinogenic potential: Some nanoparticles have been associated with an increased risk of cancer, although research is still ongoing to fully understand their carcinogenic impact.

Neurological effects: There are concerns about their ability to cross the blood-brain barrier, potentially causing neurological damage.

Environmental impact

Aquatic ecosystems: Nanoparticles can end up in aquatic ecosystems, affecting aquatic flora and fauna and disrupting food chains.

Soil and Agriculture: Their presence in the soil can affect the health of plants and the quality of agricultural produce.

Management and regulations

Monitoring and Risk Assessment: It is crucial to monitor the environment for the presence of nanoparticles and to assess their potential risks to health and the environment.

Regulations and safety standards: The development of specific regulations for the production, use and disposal of nanoparticles is necessary to minimise their impact.

Ongoing research is essential to better understand the long-term effects of nanoparticles on human health and the environment. A precautionary and prudent approach is recommended to manage the risks associated with these microscopic pollutants.

Unknown Risks in Everyday Life

In our daily lives, we are often exposed to little-known or underestimated environmental risks, which can have significant implications for our health. Here are some of these hidden risks:

Chemicals in Consumer Products

Cosmetics and Personal Care Products: Some products contain potentially harmful chemicals, such as parabens, phthalates and volatile organic compounds (VOCs).

Plastics: Plastics containing bisphenol A (BPA) or phthalates, often used in food packaging, can release these substances into food or drink.

Indoor Pollution

Indoor air quality: VOCs from paint, furniture, cleaning products and even outside air can end up inside homes, affecting indoor air quality.

Mould and dust mites: In damp or poorly ventilated environments, the growth of mould and the presence of dust mites can cause allergies and respiratory problems.

Exposure to electromagnetic fields

Electrical appliances and Wi-Fi: Continued exposure to electromagnetic fields from electrical appliances, mobile phones and Wi-Fi routers is causing concern, although the health risks remain a subject of scientific debate.

Food and Water

Pesticide residues: Non-organic fruit and vegetables may contain pesticide residues.

Contaminants in drinking water: Water can be contaminated by heavy metals, nitrates, micro-organisms and other pollutants, depending on the source and treatment of the water.

Professional life

Office environments: A sedentary lifestyle, prolonged exposure to screens and poor ergonomics at work can contribute to health problems such as musculoskeletal disorders and eye strain.

Occupational stress: Chronic work-related stress can have harmful effects on mental and physical health.

Leisure Activities

Screens and Passive Time: Excessive use of electronic devices during leisure time can contribute to a sedentary lifestyle and sleep disorders.

UV exposure during outdoor activities: Excessive exposure to the sun without adequate protection can increase the risk of skin cancer.

Raising awareness of these risks and adopting preventive measures, such as reading product labels, improving indoor air quality, using technological devices with care, and maintaining an active, healthy lifestyle, can help reduce exposure to these little-known everyday dangers.

Chapter 9

MEDICAL ADVANCES AND TECHNOLOGY

Developments in Cancer Treatment

Advances in cancer treatment in recent years have been remarkable, offering new hope and options for patients. These developments include more targeted and personalised therapies, as well as advances in technologies and treatment methods. Here are some of the significant advances:

Targeted therapies
Kinase inhibitors: These drugs block specific enzymes (kinases) involved in the growth and spread of cancer cells.
Hormonal therapy: Used mainly for breast and prostate cancers, this therapy targets the hormones that fuel the growth of certain types of cancer.
Immunotherapy
Immune checkpoint inhibitors: These drugs help the immune system to recognise and attack cancer cells.
CAR-T therapy: An advanced form of immunotherapy in which the patient's own T cells are genetically modified in the laboratory to fight cancer more effectively.
Gene and Molecular Therapies
Gene therapy: introduces genes into cancer cells or the immune system to fight or control cancer.
Blocking mRNA: Using techniques to prevent cancer cells from producing the proteins they need to grow.
Precision Medicine and Personalised Treatment
Genetic testing: Identifying specific genetic mutations in cancer cells to choose the most effective treatment.
Precision oncology: Tailoring treatment to the patient's genetic, environmental and lifestyle profile.
Advances in Radiotherapy
3D Conformal Radiotherapy: Uses 3D images to precisely target the tumour, minimising damage to surrounding healthy tissue.
Proton therapy: uses protons rather than traditional X-rays, enabling more precise targeting of the tumour with fewer side effects.
Robot-Assisted Surgery
Minimally Invasive Surgery: Using robots to perform precise surgery, reducing complications and recovery time.

Supportive Treatments and Palliative Care

Pain and Side Effect Management: Improving strategies for managing the pain and side effects of cancer treatment.

Integrated Palliative Care: Providing holistic support to patients, focusing on quality of life and emotional well-being.

These developments reflect a significant change in the approach to cancer treatment, with an increasing focus on more personalised and less invasive therapies, while improving efficacy and reducing side effects. Continued research in these areas is essential if we are to develop even more effective and accessible treatments in the future.

Innovative pollution control technologies

Innovative pollution control technologies play a crucial role in the fight against environmental pollution. These technologies aim to reduce, eliminate or transform pollutants in the air, water and soil. Here are some of the most promising innovations in this field:

Air Pollution Control

Advanced Air Purifiers: Systems using HEPA filters, activated carbon and even CO2 capture technologies to purify indoor and outdoor air.

Photocatalysis: Use of light, often in combination with catalysts such as titanium dioxide, to break down atmospheric pollutants into less harmful substances.

Biotechnologies: Use of micro-organisms or plants to absorb and break down atmospheric pollutants.

Water Treatment

Nanofiltration and Reverse Osmosis: Advanced filtration technologies to remove contaminants from water, including heavy metals and microplastics.

Phytoremediation: Use of plants to absorb and eliminate pollutants from contaminated water.

Membrane Bioreactors: Combination of biological processes and membrane filtration to treat wastewater.

Soil sanitation

Bioremediation: Use of micro-organisms to break down organic pollutants in the soil.

Phytostabilisation: Use of plants to immobilise contaminants in the soil, preventing them from spreading.

Electrokinetics: Application of electrical currents to extract pollutants from the soil.

Carbon Capture and Storage

Direct Air Capture (DAC) technologies: Systems that capture carbon dioxide directly from the ambient air.

Geological storage: Sequestration of captured CO2 in underground geological formations.

Recycling and Waste Management

Advanced Recycling: Technologies for recycling complex materials, including plastics and electronic waste.

Waste-to-Energy: Converting waste into useful energy, thereby reducing the amount of waste sent to landfill.

Renewable and Clean Energy

Development of Alternative Energy Sources: Investment in solar, wind, hydroelectric and geothermal energy to reduce dependence on fossil fuels.

These constantly evolving pollution control technologies are essential for tackling current and future environmental challenges. By combining technological innovation with political commitment, it is possible to significantly reduce the impact of pollution on the environment and human health.

Artificial Intelligence and Big Data against Cancer

Artificial intelligence (AI) and Big Data are playing an increasingly important role in the fight against cancer, offering innovative prospects for diagnosis, treatment and research. Here are some key areas where these technologies are transforming the fight against cancer:

Early Diagnosis and Detection

Medical Imaging Analysis: AI can quickly and accurately analyse medical images, such as X-rays, MRIs and CT scans, to detect tumours at an early stage.

Digital Pathology: AI helps analyse tissue samples, improving diagnostic accuracy and classifying cancer types.

Personalisation of Treatment

Precision oncology: AI can analyse tumour genetic data to identify the best treatment strategies for each patient.

Predictive models: Using patient data, AI can predict how an individual will respond to a specific treatment, enabling a more personalised approach.

Drug Research and Development

Drug design: AI accelerates the discovery of new drugs by identifying potential therapeutic targets and predicting compound efficacy.

Clinical Trials: AI helps optimise the design and management of clinical trials, improving efficiency and reducing costs.

Patient Care Management

Patient monitoring: AI-based systems can help track patient progress, manage side effects and adjust treatments in real time.

Virtual Assistance: Chatbots and virtual assistants can provide information and support to patients, improving communication and engagement.

Large-scale data analysis

Big Data in Oncology: The analysis of large cancer datasets can reveal trends, patterns and correlations that escape traditional methods of analysis.

Bioinformatics: AI and Big Data are helping to interpret complex genomic, proteomic and metabolomic data in cancer research.

Prevention and awareness

Risk models: AI can analyse demographic and clinical data to identify high-risk individuals, enabling targeted preventive interventions.

Education and awareness: Intelligent platforms can provide personalised information on cancer prevention and early detection.

AI and Big Data offer revolutionary possibilities in the fight against cancer, from the molecular and individual level to large population studies. As these technologies continue to evolve, they promise to radically transform the understanding, diagnosis, treatment and prevention of cancer.

Chapter 10

GLOBAL PERSPECTIVES AND INTERNATIONAL CASE STUDIES

International comparisons on Pollution and Cancer

International comparisons on pollution and cancer reveal significant differences in cancer incidence, types of pollutants, and public health policies across the world. These comparisons provide a better understanding of how different environmental, economic and cultural factors influence the relationship between pollution and cancer. Here are some key aspects:

Incidence of Cancer and Types of Pollution

High-income countries: In these countries, industrial and urban pollution, particularly air pollution and chemical contaminants, is often linked to higher rates of certain cancers, such as lung cancer and melanoma.

Low- and middle-income countries: These countries may face different types of pollution, such as water pollution due to poor management of industrial and household waste, which may be associated with increased rates of gastrointestinal or bladder cancer.

Public Health Policy and Legislation

Standards and regulations : Countries with strict air and water quality standards tend to have lower rates of pollution-related cancers.

Access to healthcare: The availability and quality of healthcare, including cancer screening and treatment, varies greatly and influences cancer survival rates.

Impact of Industrial and Urban Practices

Urbanisation: Countries with high levels of urbanisation may experience increased air pollution, influencing rates of lung cancer and other respiratory diseases.

Industry and agriculture: Industrial and agricultural practices, particularly the use of pesticides and chemicals, vary and have a direct impact on cancer rates in different regions.

Socio-economic and cultural factors

Inequalities: Socio-economic inequalities, both within and between countries, can lead to unequal exposure to pollution and unequal access to healthcare.

Lifestyle and Cultural Factors: Diet, lifestyle and cultural practices can interact with pollution to influence cancer rates.

International Research and Collaboration

> **Comparative studies:** International research provides valuable data on the impact of different types of pollution on health.
>
> **Exchanges of best practice:** International collaboration enables the sharing of effective strategies for reducing pollution and preventing cancer.

These international comparisons underline the importance of comprehensive and tailored approaches to managing the impact of pollution on cancer. They also provide opportunities to learn from different experiences and to implement more effective policies and interventions on a global scale.

Country Lessons
in Response to these Scourges

The responses of different countries to the scourges of pollution and cancer offer valuable lessons. These lessons, drawn from the successes and challenges encountered, can guide future strategies for better management of public health and the environment. Here are some of the key lessons:

Multifactorial approach

> **Integration of strategies:** The need to integrate environmental, public health and economic strategies to effectively address the relationship between pollution and cancer.
>
> **Intersectoral collaboration:** Collaboration between governments, non-governmental organisations, the private sector and communities is crucial to an effective response.

Importance of Prevention

> **Pollution Reduction:** Effective pollution reduction policies, such as emission standards for industry and vehicles, have a significant impact on cancer prevention.
>
> **Awareness-raising and education:** Public awareness campaigns play a key role in changing behaviour and reducing the risk of pollution-related cancer.

Innovation and Technology

> **Technological development:** Investment in pollution control technologies and support for innovative research

are essential if we are to face up to environmental and health challenges.

Use of Data and AI: The exploitation of data, including the use of artificial intelligence, can improve pollution monitoring and the early diagnosis of cancer.

Public Health Policy

Robust healthcare systems: Building healthcare systems capable of managing both cancer prevention and treatment is essential.

Screening programmes: Early detection of cancer, facilitated by accessible programmes, considerably increases survival rates.

Regulations and legislation

Strict standards: The adoption of strict environmental regulations and their effective enforcement are fundamental to reducing exposure to carcinogenic pollutants.

Evidence-based policies: Policies must be based on sound scientific data and ongoing evaluation of their effectiveness.

Community contribution

Community mobilisation: Involving communities in environmental monitoring and health awareness enhances initiatives to combat pollution and cancer.

Equity and justice: It is crucial to tackle inequalities in health and the environment, ensuring that the measures taken benefit all sections of the population equally.

By learning from the experiences of different countries, the international community can strengthen its efforts to combat pollution and reduce the incidence of cancer, while promoting healthier environments and more resilient societies.

International Cooperation and Transnational Studies

International cooperation and transnational studies are essential to effectively address pollution and cancer issues, which are global problems that know no borders. Here are some key areas where international cooperation and transnational studies play a crucial role:

Sharing Data and Resources

Data exchange: International collaboration facilitates the sharing of epidemiological and environmental data, leading to a better understanding of the links between pollution and cancer.

Research resources: Sharing resources, technologies and expertise can accelerate research and innovation in the fight against cancer and the reduction of pollution.

Transnational Studies

International comparisons: Transnational studies allow cancer incidence and pollution levels to be compared between different countries, offering unique insights into risk factors and prevention strategies.

Surveys of Specific Pollutants: Studies carried out in several countries can help identify the effects of specific pollutants on human health across different populations and environments.

International Agreements and Initiatives

Environmental agreements: Agreements such as the Paris Climate Agreement play a key role in reducing emissions of greenhouse gases and other pollutants.

Global health programmes: Initiatives such as those of the World Health Organisation (WHO) to control cancer and reduce pollution help to coordinate international efforts.

Collaboration on Public Health Policies

Setting standards: International cooperation is essential to establish global standards for air, water and food quality.

Prevention Strategies: Sharing best practice in cancer prevention and pollution management can improve public health policies worldwide.

Help and Technical Assistance

Support for developing countries: International cooperation often involves support for developing countries to improve their pollution management and health infrastructures.

Crisis Response: International collaboration is crucial to responding effectively to health and environmental emergencies, such as industrial disasters.

Global Awareness and Education

Information campaigns: International organisations can run global awareness campaigns on the risks of pollution and cancer.

Educational Programmes : Transnational educational initiatives can raise awareness and provide information on best practice in cancer prevention and environmental protection.

International cooperation and transnational studies are therefore essential for a global understanding and effective action against pollution and cancer. They enable a unified and coordinated approach, which is essential in the face of challenges that transcend national borders.

Chapter 11

HUMAN RIGHTS, ETHICS AND LEGISLATION

Impact on Vulnerable Populations

The impact of pollution and cancer on vulnerable populations is a major concern. These groups, often characterised by limited resources, lower adaptive capacity and increased exposure to risks, suffer disproportionately from the harmful consequences of environmental pollution and cancer. Here are some key aspects of this impact:

Increased Exposure to Pollutants

Living and working conditions: Low-income populations often live and work in more polluted environments, such as near factories, landfill sites or in densely populated areas with poor air quality.

Lack of access to clean water: These communities may have limited access to drinking water, exposing them to contaminants linked to cancer risks.

Reduced access to healthcare

Screening and treatment : Vulnerable populations often have less access to cancer screening services and advanced treatments.

Prevention and education: There may be a lack of information and awareness about cancer prevention and the risks associated with pollution.

Social and Economic Inequalities

Economic impact: The costs associated with cancer treatment and the loss of income due to the disease can be devastating for low-income families.

Marginalisation: Marginalised populations, including certain ethnic minorities and indigenous groups, can be particularly affected by systemic discrimination and marginalisation.

Effects on children

Development and health: Children in vulnerable communities are particularly at risk, as pollution can affect their physical and cognitive development and increase their risk of cancer in adulthood.

Impact on women

Increased risks: In certain populations, women may be more exposed to specific household or occupational pollutants, increasing their risk of certain types of cancer.

Psychological repercussions

Stress and anxiety: Living with the double burden of pollution and increased risk of illness can have a profound psychological impact, particularly in terms of stress and anxiety.

Challenges for rural and farming communities

Exposure to Pesticides: Farming communities can be exposed to pesticides and other chemicals, increasing the risk of specific cancers.

Importance of Targeted Action

Specific programmes: It is essential to set up targeted programmes for these populations, offering better access to healthcare, education and healthy environments.

Attention to the needs of vulnerable populations is crucial in the fight against pollution and cancer. This requires a comprehensive approach that takes account of social, economic and health inequalities, and aims to reduce these disparities.

Ethical Debates and Human Rights

The relationship between pollution, cancer and human rights raises important ethical debates. These discussions focus on the responsibilities of governments and companies, the rights of individuals to a healthy environment, and inequalities in exposure to risks and access to care. Here are some key aspects of these debates:

The right to a healthy environment

Fundamental human rights: Access to a clean and safe environment is increasingly recognised as a fundamental human right. Pollution that increases the risk of cancer calls this right into question.

Government responsibility: Governments have a responsibility to protect their citizens from environmental hazards and to regulate polluting activities.

Environmental Justice

Inequalities in exposure: Poor communities and minorities are often more exposed to pollution, which raises questions of environmental justice.

Access to healthcare: Inequal access to cancer screening and treatment is also a major health justice issue.

Corporate Responsibility

Industrial pollution: Companies are often at the centre of debate because of their role in environmental pollution. Their responsibility towards society and the environment is widely debated.

Transparency and accountability: There is a growing demand for companies to be transparent about their environmental impact and to be held accountable for any damage caused.

Sustainable development

Balancing Growth and the Environment: How can societies balance economic growth with environmental protection and public health?

Sustainability Principles: Discussions focus on the adoption of sustainable development practices to reduce pollution and prevent cancer.

Informed Consent and Patients' Rights

Risk information: Individuals have the right to be informed about the environmental and health risks associated with their living and working environment.

Health Decisions: Patients have the right to make informed decisions about their cancer treatment, based on full and accessible information.

Research ethics

Experimentation and testing: the ethical issues surrounding the testing of new cancer treatments, including the use of animals and the consent of human participants.

Research priorities: What should be the research priorities, taking into account both global needs and commercial interests?

These ethical debates and human rights issues are essential in guiding policy and practice in environmental health and cancer control. They underline the importance of a balanced approach that respects the rights of individuals while pursuing public and environmental health objectives.

Legal frameworks and liability of Companies

Legal frameworks and corporate responsibility play a crucial role in pollution management and cancer prevention. They establish the rules, standards and obligations that govern the way companies operate, particularly with regard to their impact on the environment and human health. Here are some important aspects of these frameworks:

Environmental legislation

Pollution standards: Environmental laws set standards for air, water and soil quality, limiting the levels of harmful pollutants.

Industrial emissions: Specific regulations control emissions from factories, power stations and other industrial sources to minimise their impact on public health.

Corporate Responsibility

Corporate Social Responsibility (CSR): There is a growing expectation that companies should act responsibly, not only towards their shareholders, but also towards society and the environment.

Precautionary principle: Companies are encouraged to adopt preventive approaches to minimise environmental and health risks.

Environmental and Health Law

Toxic Substances Regulations: Laws regulate the use and management of potentially hazardous chemical substances to reduce exposure of workers and the public.

Right to information: Regulations such as the right to environmental information give citizens access to data on pollution and health risks.

Legal action

Class actions: Individuals affected by pollution can join together to bring collective actions against the companies responsible for the contamination.

Damages: Companies may be required to pay damages for health impacts caused by their polluting activities.

International agreements

Cross-border cooperation: International agreements, such as the Paris Climate Agreement, play an important role in managing global environmental issues.

Global Standards: These agreements help to establish global standards for the management of pollutants and the protection of public health.

Monitoring and Compliance

Inspections and audits: Government agencies carry out inspections and audits to ensure that companies comply with environmental standards.

Transparency and reporting: Companies are increasingly required to report on their environmental impact and their efforts to reduce it.

The effectiveness of these legal frameworks and corporate responsibility depends on their rigorous implementation and an ongoing commitment to improving environmental practices. This requires collaboration between governments, businesses, non-governmental organisations and citizens to create a healthier environment and reduce the risk of pollution-related cancer.

Chapter 12

EDUCATION AND AWARENESS

The role of education in prevention

Education plays a fundamental role in preventing pollution and cancer. It is essential to raise awareness, inform and empower individuals and communities to take proactive steps to protect their health and their environment. Here are some key aspects of the role of education in this context:

Raising awareness and providing information

Understanding the risks: Education helps people to understand the risks associated with pollution and how it can contribute to the development of cancer.

Promotion of Healthy Behaviours: Educational programmes can encourage behaviours and lifestyle habits that reduce the risk of cancer, such as adopting a healthy diet, regular exercise and avoiding smoking.

Education in Schools

Integration into school curricula: Introducing subjects related to the environment, public health and cancer prevention into school curricula can raise awareness among the younger generation from an early age.

Educational activities and projects: School projects that focus on the environment, such as science clubs, school gardens and recycling projects, can increase pupils' awareness and commitment.

Training and Resources for Healthcare Professionals

Medical training: Training health professionals on the links between pollution, the environment and cancer so that they can better advise and treat their patients.

Resources and Educational Material: Providing healthcare professionals with resources to educate their patients about cancer prevention and pollution-related risks.

Public awareness campaigns

Awareness programmes: Using the media, poster campaigns and social networks to disseminate information about the dangers of pollution and ways of reducing the risk of cancer.

Theme Days: Organising events and campaigns around global days, such as World Environment Day or World Cancer Day, to raise public awareness.

Community contribution

Workshops and Seminars: Organise community workshops to discuss local pollution and health problems, and to share prevention strategies.

Community Mobilisation: Encouraging the active participation of communities in environmental and health initiatives.

Use of Modern Technologies

Online tools and applications: Use online platforms and mobile applications to provide accessible information on pollution and cancer prevention.

Interactive Educational Programmes: Developing interactive educational programmes and games to raise awareness in an engaging way.

Education is therefore a powerful tool for preventing pollution and cancer, offering the opportunity to inform, empower and engage individuals and communities at all levels. By investing in education, societies can foster greater awareness and more effective action for health and the environment.

Community Awareness Programmes

Community awareness programmes are essential for informing and mobilising people around the issues of pollution and cancer prevention. These programmes can take various forms and be adapted to the specific needs of each community. Here are some effective examples of awareness-raising programmes:

Workshops and Educational Seminars

Awareness-raising themes: Organising workshops on the effects of pollution on health, ways of reducing exposure to pollutants, and cancer prevention strategies.

Experts and Speakers: Invite health professionals, environmental experts and cancer survivors to talk about their experiences and knowledge.

Public awareness campaigns

Use of the media: Disseminate awareness-raising messages through local media, including television, radio and social networks.

Informative material: Distribute brochures, posters and leaflets in public places, schools and health centres.

School programmes
> **Environmental education:** integrating education on pollution and health into school curricula.
> **Student projects:** Encourage student projects focusing on the environment and health, such as science fairs and environmental clubs.

Community Involvement and Mobilisation
> **Community Clean-ups:** Organising clean-up events to raise awareness of local pollution and promote a clean environment.
> **Community gardens:** Creating community gardens to encourage healthy eating and raise awareness of sustainable agriculture.

Working with healthcare professionals
> **Screening clinics:** Offer cancer screening clinics in community centres to facilitate access to health services.
> **Training health professionals:** training community health workers to raise awareness of cancer and pollution.

Using Technology
> **Mobile applications:** Developing applications providing information on local air quality, health advice and cancer screening resources.
> **Online platforms:** Using online platforms to create virtual support communities and share information.

Special Events and Activities
> **Walks and Runs:** Organise walks or runs to raise awareness of cancer and raise funds for research and patient support.
> **Theme Days:** Celebrating global days, such as World Environment Day or World Cancer Day, with educational activities and events.

These programmes can make a major contribution to raising collective awareness of pollution and cancer issues, while strengthening community cohesion and encouraging positive action for health and the environment.

Mobilising young people
for the Environment and Health

Mobilising young people for environmental and health causes is crucial, because young people are not only the inheritors of our planet, but also influential agents of change. Here are some strategies for effectively engaging young people in these areas:

Education and awareness-raising in schools

Educational programmes: Incorporate lessons on the environment, sustainability and health into school curricula to raise awareness from an early age.

Projects and Activities: Encourage school projects focusing on the environment, such as ecological gardens, recycling campaigns and scientific projects on pollution.

Social Media Platforms

Use of Social Networks: Use social media platforms to share information, inspiring stories and opportunities for engagement with young people.

Influencers and Ambassadors: Working with young influencers to promote messages about the environment and health.

Leadership and Volunteering Programmes

Youth Leadership Programmes: Creating programmes that enable young people to develop skills in leadership and in managing environmental and health projects.

Volunteering opportunities: Offering volunteering opportunities in environmental and health organisations to enable young people to play an active part in these causes.

Targeted campaigns and events

Engaging events: Organise events such as conferences, workshops, competitions and green marathons that are attractive and informative for young people.

Awareness campaigns: Launch campaigns focusing on themes that resonate with young people, such as climate change, plastic pollution and healthy living.

Working with universities and colleges

Research and Innovation: Encouraging research and innovation in the fields of the environment and health within educational institutions.

Clubs and societies: Support the formation of student clubs and societies focusing on the environment and health.

Use of Technology and Applications

Educational applications: Developing applications and games that teach the principles of sustainability, pollution management and cancer prevention in a fun and engaging way.

Collaborative platforms: Creating online platforms for collaboration, sharing ideas and initiating environmental and health projects.

Encouragement of local initiatives

Community projects: Encouraging young people to get involved in environmental and health projects in their communities.

Mentoring and networking: Set up mentoring programmes and support networks to guide young people in their initiatives.

By mobilising young people, not only are we preparing a future generation that is aware and responsible, but we are also benefiting from their energy, creativity and ability to have a positive influence on society.

Chapter 13

INDUSTRIAL POLLUTION AND OCCUPATIONAL CANCER

Carcinogenic risks in Industrial Environments

Industrial environments present specific carcinogenic risks due to exposure to various chemical, physical and biological agents. Here are some of the carcinogenic risks commonly associated with these environments:

Exposure to Chemical Agents
Asbestos: Used in the past for insulation and construction products, asbestos is a well-known carcinogen, linked to mesothelioma and lung cancer.
Benzene: Found in crude oil and petroleum products, benzene is associated with leukaemia.
Formaldehyde: Used in the manufacture of pressed wood products, resins and textiles, formaldehyde is linked to nasopharyngeal cancers and leukaemia.
Polycyclic Aromatic Hydrocarbons (PAHs): Generated during the incomplete combustion of organic matter, PAHs are associated with cancers of the skin, lungs, bladder and gastrointestinal tract.
Physical agents
Ionising radiation: Exposure to ionising radiation, such as that encountered in the nuclear industry, can increase the risk of various cancers, including leukaemia and thyroid cancer.
Dust and particles: In industries such as mining, inhalation of fine dust can lead to lung cancer.
Biological factors
Exposure to infectious agents: Certain industrial environments, particularly in agriculture and food processing, can expose workers to infectious agents that increase the risk of cancer.
Physical and Thermal Stress
Extreme heat and cold: Working in conditions of extreme heat or cold can indirectly increase the risk of certain types of cancer.
Prevention and safety measures
Personal Protective Equipment: Provide and require the use of suitable protective equipment to minimise exposure to carcinogenic substances.
Training and awareness: Educating workers about the risks associated with their work environment and safe working practices.

Controls and regulations: Implementing strict controls on the use of carcinogenic substances and ensuring compliance with workplace safety regulations.

Worker Health Monitoring: Carrying out regular medical examinations and exposure assessments to detect any signs of illness linked to the work environment at an early stage.

It is crucial that companies and regulators work together to identify and manage these risks, thereby protecting the health of workers and helping to prevent cancer in industrial environments.

Case Studies on Occupational Illnesses Linked to Pollution

Pollution-related occupational illnesses are an important subject for study, as they highlight the consequences of exposure to harmful working environments. Here are a few emblematic case studies:

1. Lung diseases in coal mines

   Context: Coal miners are exposed to coal dust, which can lead to chronic lung diseases such as coal miners' pneumoconiosis (CWP), also known as "black lung".

   Consequences: Prolonged exposure can cause serious lung damage and increase the risk of chronic respiratory disease and lung cancer.

2. Mesothelioma in workers exposed to asbestos

   Background: Exposure to asbestos, common in the construction and ship-repair industries and in the manufacture of insulation products, is linked to mesothelioma, an aggressive cancer of the pleura.

   Impact: Workers exposed to asbestos can develop this disease several decades after their first exposure, underlining the insidious nature of the risk.

3. Skin cancers in farmers

   Background: Farmers, who spend long hours in the sun, are at increased risk of skin cancers such as basal cell carcinoma and melanoma.

Prevention: This situation has led to initiatives to raise awareness of the importance of sun protection and regular skin checks.

4. Leukaemia in the chemical industry

Background: Workers in the chemical industry exposed to substances such as benzene are at increased risk of acute leukaemia.

Safety measures: These cases have reinforced the need for strict safety standards and personal protection measures in the industry.

5. Respiratory disorders in the textile industry

Context: Workers in textile factories, particularly those involved in cotton production, can develop byssinosis, a respiratory disease linked to the inhalation of cotton dust.

Solutions: Improving ventilation and providing respiratory protection equipment are key measures for reducing this risk.

6. Radiation-related cancers in the nuclear industry

Context: Workers in the nuclear industry exposed to high levels of ionising radiation can develop various types of cancer, particularly of the thyroid and blood.

Risk Management: This has led to strict regulation of radiation exposure and regular health checks.

These case studies highlight the importance of strict regulations, increased awareness and enhanced safety measures to prevent pollution-related occupational illnesses. They also highlight the need for ongoing monitoring of workers' health in high-risk industries.

Prevention and regulations in the Industrial Sector

Prevention and regulation in the industrial sector are essential to protect the health of workers and minimise the environmental impact of industrial activities. Here are some key strategies and regulatory practices:

Occupational health and safety standards

Personal Protective Equipment (PPE): Providing and requiring the use of appropriate PPE, such as masks, gloves and protective clothing, to reduce exposure to hazardous substances.

Safety training: Provide regular training to employees on safe working practices, the correct use of PPE and emergency management.

Environmental Controls

Ventilation Systems: Installing and maintaining effective ventilation systems to reduce exposure to airborne pollutants in working environments.

Emissions Reduction: Implementing technologies and processes that reduce emissions of pollutants into the air, water and soil.

Regulations and Legislative Standards

Compliance with Standards: Ensuring that all industrial operations comply with the environmental and workplace safety standards established by local and international legislation.

Audits and Inspections: Conducting regular audits and inspections to ensure compliance with safety and environmental standards.

Worker Health Monitoring

Regular medical examinations: Offer regular medical examinations to employees to detect the harmful effects of exposure to hazardous substances at an early stage.

Surveillance programmes: Set up health surveillance programmes to monitor trends and patterns of work-related illness.

Waste and Chemicals Management

Safe storage: Ensure the safe storage of chemical substances to prevent leaks, spills and accidental exposure.

Responsible disposal: Managing the disposal of industrial waste in an environmentally-friendly way to reduce the impact on the environment.

Sustainable Development and Social Responsibility

Sustainable Practices: Adopting sustainable business practices to minimise environmental impact.

Community Involvement: Working with local communities to address environmental and health concerns.

Innovation and Continuous Improvement

Research and Development: Investing in the research and development of cleaner, safer technologies.

Process Improvement: Encouraging the continuous improvement of processes to increase efficiency while reducing environmental and health risks.

By adopting these measures, the industrial sector can play a crucial role in preventing pollution-related illnesses, including cancer, and contribute to a more sustainable and healthier future.

Chapter 14

TECHNOLOGY AT YOUR SERVICE OF ENVIRONMENT

Innovations in Pollution Monitoring

Innovations in pollution monitoring are essential for detecting, measuring and analysing environmental pollutants. These advanced technologies enable more effective and accurate monitoring, helping to prevent harmful impacts on human health and the environment. Here are some notable examples of innovations in this field:

Sensors and Monitoring Stations
Air Quality Sensors: Advanced sensors can measure specific pollutants in the air, such as fine particles (PM2.5), nitrogen dioxide and ozone.
Environmental Monitoring Stations: Stations equipped with multiple sensors provide real-time data on air, water and soil quality.
Satellite and Airborne Technologies
Satellite imagery: The use of satellites to monitor greenhouse gas emissions, deforestation and atmospheric pollutants on a large scale.
Drones: The use of sensor-equipped drones to collect data on pollutants in hard-to-reach areas.
Big Data and Artificial Intelligence
Big Data Analysis: The use of Big Data to analyse large volumes of environmental data and detect trends and patterns.
Predictive models: The application of artificial intelligence to predict pollution levels and their potential impact on health and the environment.
Mobile Applications and Online Platforms
Air Quality Applications: Mobile applications provide citizens with real-time information on air quality, enabling them to make informed decisions about their health.
Crowdsourcing platforms: Online platforms where citizens can report and share data on local pollution.
Portable and Personal Sensor Networks
Portable Sensors: Portable devices that individuals can use to monitor their personal exposure to various pollutants.
Intelligent clothing: Integrating sensors into clothing to monitor exposure to pollution continuously and discreetly.

Water and Soil Analysis
> **Water Test Kits:** Portable kits for testing water quality, detecting contaminants such as heavy metals, nitrates and bacteria.
>
> **Soil analysers:** devices for assessing soil contamination and monitoring the health of terrestrial ecosystems.

These innovations not only improve our ability to monitor and understand pollution, they also help governments, businesses and individuals to take proactive measures to reduce it and protect public health.

Purification Systems and Advanced Filtration

Advanced purification and filtration systems play a crucial role in reducing pollution and protecting public health. These technologies are essential for eliminating or reducing the presence of contaminants in air, water and other environments. Here are a few noteworthy innovations in this field:

Air Purification
> **HEPA (High-Efficiency Particulate Air) filters:** These filters are extremely effective at capturing fine particles, including allergens, mould spores and smoke particles.
>
> **Air Purifiers with UV Technology:** Use ultraviolet light to destroy bacteria, viruses and other micro-organisms.
>
> **Ionisation Air Purifiers:** Capture pollutant particles by electrically charging them.

Water Filtration
> **Reverse osmosis:** This technique uses a semi-permeable membrane to remove ions, unwanted molecules and larger particles from the water.
>
> **Activated carbon filters:** Eliminate organic contaminants, chlorine and bad tastes and odours from water.
>
> **Biofiltration systems:** Use natural materials or micro-organisms to filter contaminants from water.

Purification of the Indoor Environment
> **Intelligent Ventilation Systems:** These systems actively control indoor air quality, adjusting ventilation according to the pollution levels detected.

Indoor plants: Certain plants are known for their ability to filter atmospheric pollutants and can be used as a natural means of purifying the air.

Nanotechnology technology

Nanotechnology-based filters: These filters use nanomaterials to capture specific pollutants at a molecular level, providing extremely fine filtration.

Waste Water Treatment Systems

Advanced wastewater treatment technologies: Systems such as membrane bioreactors and sand filtration treat wastewater before it is released into the environment.

Industrial wastewater treatment: specialised treatment of industrial wastewater to remove specific pollutants such as heavy metals and toxic chemical compounds.

Purification in Emergency Situations

Portable Systems: Portable water filtration units for emergency situations, capable of transforming contaminated water into drinking water.

These advanced purification and filtration technologies are essential for protecting public health and the environment from the harmful effects of pollution. Their continued development is crucial to meeting the growing challenges posed by pollution in the modern world.

The Impact of Green Technology on Cancer Risk Reduction

Green technology is playing a significant role in reducing the risk of cancer by addressing environmental issues related to pollution. Here are some key areas where green technology can have a positive impact:

Renewable Energy

Reducing greenhouse gas emissions: The use of renewable energies, such as wind, solar and hydroelectric power, reduces dependence on fossil fuels, thereby cutting emissions of carcinogenic atmospheric pollutants.

Improved air quality: Better air quality resulting from the use of clean energy can significantly reduce the risk of lung cancer and other respiratory diseases.

Electric Vehicles and Sustainable Transport
> **Reducing vehicle emissions:** Electric vehicles and sustainable modes of transport, such as cycling and public transport, reduce air pollution in urban areas.
>
> **Less noise pollution: In** addition to air pollution, reducing traffic noise can also have beneficial effects on overall health.

Green Buildings
> **Eco-friendly Building Materials:** Using non-toxic, eco-friendly materials in construction reduces exposure to hazardous chemicals in indoor environments.
>
> **Efficient energy management:** Green buildings designed for greater energy efficiency also help to reduce overall emissions of pollutants.

Sustainable Agriculture
> **Reducing the use of pesticides:** Organic farming and sustainable agricultural practices limit exposure to pesticides, which are linked to certain types of cancer.
>
> **Preserving water quality:** Sustainable farming techniques help to prevent the contamination of groundwater and watercourses.

Pollution Control Technologies
> **Air and Water Purification:** Advanced filtration and purification technologies remove carcinogenic contaminants from air and water.
>
> **Waste management and recycling:** More environmentally-friendly waste management methods reduce the release of toxic substances into the environment.

Awareness-raising and education
> **Awareness-raising programmes:** Green technology, accompanied by educational programmes, increases public awareness of the links between the environment and health, including the risks of cancer.

By adopting green technology and promoting sustainable practices, it is possible to significantly reduce the environmental risk factors for cancer. This transition towards greener solutions is essential not only for human health, but also for the overall health of our planet.

Chapter 15

FOOD, POLLUTION AND CANCER

Impact of Pesticides and Chemicals in Agriculture

The use of pesticides and chemical products in agriculture has a significant impact on human health and the environment. Although these products are essential for controlling pests and increasing agricultural productivity, there are a number of risks associated with their use:

Risks to human health

Direct exposure: Farmers and agricultural workers who handle pesticides may be directly exposed, increasing their risk of developing chronic diseases, including certain types of cancer.

Residues in food: Pesticide residues on fruit, vegetables and cereals can pose risks to consumers. Some pesticides have been linked to various health problems, including cancer, neurological disorders and reproductive problems.

Water contamination: Pesticides can seep into groundwater and contaminate drinking water sources, posing health risks for remote populations.

Impact on the environment

Loss of biodiversity: Pesticides can kill non-target species such as beneficial insects, birds and aquatic organisms, reducing biodiversity.

Surface water pollution: Pesticide run-off from agricultural fields can contaminate rivers, lakes and streams, affecting aquatic ecosystems.

Pesticide resistance: Excessive use of pesticides can lead to resistance in pest species, necessitating the use of even more powerful and toxic products.

Alternatives and Solutions

Organic farming: Organic farming uses natural methods to combat pests and diseases, reducing dependence on chemical products.

Low-risk pesticides: The development and use of low-risk, biodegradable pesticides can minimise negative impacts.

Integrated Pest Management (IPM): IPM combines different pest management strategies to reduce dependence on chemical pesticides.

Education and training: Training farmers in sustainable farming practices and the safe use of pesticides.

Regulation and supervision

Regulatory controls: Governments impose strict regulations on the approval, use and management of pesticides.

Residue monitoring: Food residue monitoring programmes help to ensure that pesticide levels remain within established safety limits.

The impact of pesticides and chemicals in agriculture is a complex issue requiring a balance between the benefits of their use in food production and the potential risks to human health and the environment. Ongoing efforts are needed to develop safer and more sustainable farming practices.

The role of food in Cancer Prevention

Diet plays a crucial role in cancer prevention. A great deal of research shows that certain foods and eating habits can reduce the risk of developing certain types of cancer. Here are the main aspects of the role of diet in cancer prevention:

Consumption of fruit and vegetables

- **Rich in nutrients:** Fruit and vegetables are rich in vitamins, minerals, fibre and antioxidants, which can help protect against cancer.
- **Phytochemicals:** They contain phytochemicals, compounds that have been linked to a reduced risk of several types of cancer.

Balanced Diet

- **Dietary diversity:** A varied diet that includes plenty of fruit and vegetables, whole grains and lean proteins can help reduce the risk of cancer.
- **Limiting saturated and trans fats:** Reducing consumption of saturated and trans fats, found in processed foods and red meat, is also recommended for cancer prevention.

Reducing consumption of red and processed meat

- **Increased risk:** Studies have shown that high consumption of red and processed meat can increase the risk of certain cancers, particularly colorectal cancer.
- **Healthy alternatives:** Favour lean protein sources such as poultry, fish, legumes and nuts.

Alcohol and Cancer

- **Alcohol Risk:** Excessive alcohol consumption has been linked to an increased risk of several types of cancer, including liver, breast and oesophageal cancer.
- **Moderation or abstinence:** Limiting alcohol consumption or abstaining from alcohol can help reduce the risk of cancer.

Body weight and diet

- **Obesity and cancer:** Overweight and obesity are risk factors for several types of cancer. A balanced diet, combined with physical exercise, is essential for maintaining a healthy weight.
- **Diet and physical activity:** Adopting a healthy diet and being physically active are two of the most important strategies for preventing cancer.

Supplements and Cancer

- **Food supplements:** There is no conclusive evidence that food supplements can reduce the risk of cancer. A balanced diet is generally preferable.

Organic food

- **Pesticides and Cancer:** Although research is still ongoing, eating organic food may reduce exposure to pesticide residues and hormones used in conventional farming.

It is important to note that no single food or diet can guarantee the prevention of cancer, but a healthy, balanced diet can play a significant role in reducing the risk. Combining good eating habits with other healthy behaviours, such as stopping smoking and regular physical activity, increases the effectiveness of prevention even further.

Bioaccumulation and food chains

Bioaccumulation and its impact on food chains is a major environmental problem, with potential repercussions for human health and ecosystems. Here are some key aspects of this phenomenon:

What is bioaccumulation?
- **Definition:** Bioaccumulation occurs when toxic chemical substances, such as heavy metals, pesticides or persistent organic pollutants (POPs), accumulate in living organisms in concentrations greater than those present in their environment.
- **Process:** These toxic substances are often poorly biodegradable and gradually accumulate in living tissue over time.

Biomagnification in food chains
- **Accumulation along the food chain:** When small contaminated organisms are eaten by larger predators, the pollutants accumulate and concentrate at each level of the food chain, a process known as biomagnification.
- **Impacts on predators at the top of the food chain:** Animals at the top of the food chain, including humans, are particularly vulnerable to the accumulation of high levels of toxins.

Effects on human health
- **Dietary exposure:** Humans can be exposed to these toxins by eating contaminated animal products, such as fish and seafood.
- **Health risks:** Long-term exposure to these pollutants can increase the risk of health problems, including the development of certain cancers, nervous system disorders, reproductive and developmental problems, and endocrine disruption.

Environmental consequences
- **Effects on wildlife:** Wild animals, particularly those in aquatic ecosystems, may suffer adverse effects such as reproductive disorders, developmental abnormalities and population decline due to bioaccumulation.
- **Ecosystem disruption:** The bioaccumulation of toxic substances can disrupt the ecological balance, affecting biodiversity and the functioning of ecosystems.

Management and prevention strategies
- **Pollutant Control:** Implementing strict regulations to control the release of hazardous substances into the environment.

- **Environmental Monitoring:** Carrying out regular checks on pollutant levels in ecosystems, particularly in high-risk areas.
- **Awareness-raising and education:** Informing the public and industry about the dangers of bioaccumulation and promoting environmentally-friendly practices.
- **Scientific research:** Carry out research to gain a better understanding of bioaccumulation processes and develop methods to reduce their impact.

Effective management of bioaccumulation is crucial to protecting human health and preserving the health of ecosystems. This requires a coordinated approach involving regulation, research, environmental monitoring and public education.

Chapter 16

PSYCHOSOCIAL ASPECTS AND CULTURAL

Cultural Perception of Pollution and Cancer

Cultural perceptions of pollution and cancer vary considerably from one society to another, influenced by historical, socio-economic, educational and media factors. These perceptions influence how individuals and communities understand, react to and manage these issues. Here are some key aspects:

Awareness and understanding
- **Level of knowledge:** In some cultures there may be a strong awareness of the dangers of pollution and its links to cancer, while in others this knowledge may be limited due to restricted access to information.
- **Myths and beliefs:** Cultural beliefs and myths can sometimes influence the perception of cancer and pollution, sometimes minimising the risks or attributing the disease to non-scientific causes.

Attitudes towards the environment and health
- **Environmental priorities:** In some societies, environmental protection and public health are major priorities, while in others, economic development may take precedence.
- **Traditional practices:** Traditional approaches to health and medicine can influence the way people perceive and treat cancer.

Influence of the Media and Education
- **Media coverage:** The media play a crucial role in shaping public perceptions of pollution and cancer, influencing awareness and understanding of the risks.
- **Education:** Education systems that integrate environmental health and cancer awareness contribute to better understanding and more effective responses.

Impact of Social Norms and Values
- **Social norms:** Cultural attitudes towards illness, death and well-being can influence the way communities approach cancer prevention and treatment.
- **Cultural values:** Values such as community solidarity, respect for nature and priority for economic growth can shape responses to pollution and cancer.

Role of Leaders and Institutions
- **Influence of Leaders:** Religious, community and political leaders can have a significant impact on public perceptions and policies relating to pollution and cancer.

- **Institutions and policies:** Political and institutional frameworks also reflect and shape cultural attitudes towards these issues.

Community and Individual Responses
- **Prevention practices:** Cultural practices in terms of diet, lifestyle and traditional medicine can influence cancer prevention strategies.
- **Responses to environmental policies:** Acceptance and support for environmental policies are also shaped by cultural factors.

By understanding the diverse cultural perceptions of pollution and cancer, policy-makers, health professionals and campaigners can develop more effective and culturally sensitive communication and intervention strategies. This is essential to promote sustainable behaviour change and improve public and environmental health.

Psychological impact on Affected Populations

The psychological impact of pollution and cancer on affected populations is profound and multifaceted. Individuals and communities confronted with these problems can experience a range of emotions and mental repercussions. Here are some key aspects of this psychological impact:

Stress and Anxiety
- **Fear of illness:** The fear of developing cancer as a result of exposure to pollution can cause significant anxiety.
- **Uncertainty and concern:** Uncertainty about the long-term effects of pollution and concern for the health of future generations can also be sources of stress.

Impact on Quality of Life
- **Lifestyle modification:** Concerns about pollution can force people to modify their lifestyle, such as avoiding certain outdoor activities, which can affect their well-being.
- **Social isolation:** People with cancer or living in heavily polluted areas may feel socially isolated or stigmatised.

Emotional repercussions
- **Emotional distress:** The diagnosis of cancer or the realisation of living in a polluted environment can cause emotional distress, including sadness, anger and despair.

- **Feeling of powerlessness:** Feeling powerless or fatalistic in the face of environmental pollution or cancer can have a negative impact on mental health.

Impact on Families and Communities

- **Family stress:** The diagnosis of cancer in a family member can lead to family stress, affecting relationships and family dynamics.
- **Community cohesion:** Communities affected by pollution or high levels of cancer may experience a sense of loss of cohesion or distrust towards the authorities and industry.

Depression and Mental Disorders

- **Increased risks:** People living in polluted areas or those suffering from cancer are more likely to experience depression and other mental disorders.
- **Need for psychological support:** It is crucial to provide adequate psychological support to these individuals and communities.

Activism and resilience

- **Community mobilisation:** In the face of pollution and cancer, certain communities can develop resilience by mobilising for collective action and environmental change.
- **Empowerment:** Activism and participation in initiatives for change can also bring a sense of empowerment and hope.

Taking account of the psychological impact of pollution and cancer is essential if we are to offer comprehensive support to the people and communities affected. This includes not only medical and environmental care, but also appropriate psychological and social support.

The role of the media and information in Awareness

The role of the media and information in raising awareness of pollution and cancer is crucial. They serve as essential platforms for educating the public, influencing public opinion and stimulating political and individual action. Here are some key aspects of this role:

Dissemination of Reliable Information

- **Public education:** The media play an important role in disseminating reliable and accessible information on the causes, effects and prevention of pollution and cancer.
- **Clarifying the Facts:** They help to demystify complex scientific information and clarify false information or myths surrounding pollution and cancer.

Awareness and Prevention

- **Awareness campaigns:** The media can launch or support awareness campaigns that highlight the problems of pollution and cancer, encourage preventive behaviour and promote healthy lifestyles.
- **Stories and testimonials:** Presenting personal stories and testimonials can make the subject more relatable and urgent for the public.

Surveillance and Criticism

- **Monitoring Government Action:** The media play a watchdog role in holding governments and companies to account for their actions on pollution and health policy.
- **Criticism and Analysis:** They provide a platform for criticising and analysing public policies, industry initiatives and environmental trends.

Platform for Debate and Discussion

- **Discussion forums:** The media provide forums where experts, decision-makers, activists and citizens can discuss pollution and cancer problems and their solutions.
- **Diversity of Opinions:** They present a range of perspectives, contributing to a balanced and informed public debate.

Influencing Policies and Behaviour

- **Policy direction:** Media coverage can influence the policy agenda by highlighting specific issues and exerting pressure for change.
- **Behaviour change:** Increased awareness can lead to changes in people's behaviour and lifestyle choices, thereby helping to prevent cancer.

Use of New Technologies

- **Social media:** Social media platforms enable information to be disseminated quickly and widely, and encourage public involvement and participation.
- **Multimedia content:** The use of various formats, such as videos, podcasts and infographics, can make information more attractive and understandable.

The media's role in raising awareness of pollution and cancer is therefore multidimensional, combining education, monitoring, debate and influence. Responsible and informed media coverage is essential to guide public opinion and support efforts to prevent and manage these issues.

Chapter 17

INVOLVEMENT AND RESPONSIBILITY OF COMPANIES

Case studies on Corporate Social Responsibility

Corporate Social Responsibility (CSR) is a key concept in contemporary business, reflecting companies' commitment to society and the environment. Specific case studies illustrate how some companies are integrating CSR into their activities, with significant impacts on public health, the environment and communities. Here are a few examples:

1. Sustainability Initiatives in the Technology Industry
   - **Case study:** Major technology companies commit to using 100% renewable energy for their operations, thereby reducing their carbon footprint.
   - **Impact:** These actions contribute to the fight against climate change and encourage the development of sustainable energy technologies.
2. Health and Safety Programmes in the Industrial Sector
   - **Case study:** Industrial companies implement rigorous health and safety programmes to protect their employees, reducing exposure to toxic substances and improving working conditions.
   - **Impact:** These measures reduce the risk of occupational illnesses, including cancer, and improve workers' quality of life.
3. Support for local communities by extractive companies
   - **Case study:** Some mining and oil companies invest in local communities by supporting education, health and infrastructure.
   - **Impact:** These investments contribute to the economic and social development of communities affected by extractive activities.
4. Green Product Policies in the Retail Sector
   - **Case study:** Retailers commit to eliminating hazardous chemicals from their products and promoting environmentally-friendly alternatives.
   - **Impact:** This reduces consumer exposure to potentially harmful substances and encourages more sustainable consumption patterns.
5. Sustainable Resource Management in the Agri-Food Sector
   - **Case study:** Agri-food companies adopt sustainable farming practices, such as reducing pesticide use and improving water management.

- **Impact:** These practices reduce the environmental impact of agriculture and improve food safety and quality.

6. Commitment to Transparency and Ethics
- **Case study:** Companies are committing to greater transparency by publishing detailed reports on their environmental and social impacts.
- **Impact:** This transparency strengthens consumer and investor confidence and stimulates continuous improvement in business practices.

These case studies show that CSR can be a powerful driver of positive change, not only for companies themselves, but also for society and the environment as a whole. By assuming their social responsibility, companies can play a key role in resolving contemporary challenges such as pollution, climate change and environmentally-related diseases such as cancer.

Regulations and Pressures
for Cleaner Production

Regulations and pressure for cleaner production play a crucial role in reducing the environmental impact of industrial and commercial activities. Here are some key aspects of these regulations and pressures:

Environmental regulations
- **Emission standards:** Strict regulations on the emission of pollutants into the air, water and soil are forcing industries to adopt cleaner technologies.
- **Use of Resources:** Laws aimed at more efficient and sustainable use of natural resources, including water and energy, encourage environmentally friendly production.
- **Waste management:** Regulations on the management and disposal of industrial waste aim to reduce pollution and promote recycling and recovery.

Market and consumer pressure
- **Demand for eco-friendly products:** Growing consumer awareness is leading to a preference for eco-friendly products, pushing companies to adopt more sustainable practices.
- **Ecological standards and labels:** Labels such as "organic", "eco-responsible" or "fair trade" influence

consumer choices and encourage companies to improve their production processes.

Sustainable Development Initiatives

- **Corporate Social Responsibility (CSR):** Companies adopt CSR policies to integrate sustainable practices into their operations and strengthen their brand image.
- **Sustainable investment:** The increase in investment in companies that follow sustainable development principles puts pressure on all companies to improve their environmental performance.

International Agreements and Initiatives

- **Environmental agreements:** Agreements such as the Paris Climate Agreement encourage countries and industries to reduce their greenhouse gas emissions.
- **International cooperation:** Collaboration between countries to establish international environmental standards puts additional pressure on companies to comply with these standards.

Technology and Innovation

- **Development of Green Technologies:** Innovation in clean technologies offers companies more efficient and less polluting options.
- **Subsidies and Tax Incentives:** Government incentives for the adoption of clean technologies help companies make the transition to more sustainable practices.

Pressure from Shareholders and Investors

- **Responsible Investment:** Shareholders and investors are putting increasing pressure on companies to adopt sustainable practices to minimise risk and ensure long-term viability.

By combining strict regulations, market pressures, sustainable development initiatives and technological innovation, it is possible to encourage a transition towards cleaner, more environmentally-friendly production. This transition is essential to reduce the impact of industrial activities on human health and the planet.

Sustainable Innovations in the Private Sector

The private sector plays a key role in promoting sustainable innovation, with many companies adopting and developing technologies and practices that reduce environmental impact while supporting economic growth. Here are some examples of sustainable innovation in the private sector:

Renewable Energy and Energy Efficiency
- **Development of solar and wind technologies:** Companies are investing in advanced solar technologies and more efficient wind turbines to increase the production of renewable energy.
- **High Energy Efficiency Buildings:** Construction of commercial and industrial buildings using environmentally-friendly materials and innovative designs to reduce energy consumption.

Sustainable mobility
- **Electric and hybrid vehicles:** Car manufacturers are investing in the development of electric and hybrid vehicles to reduce greenhouse gas emissions.
- **Shared Mobility Solutions:** Transport companies are developing shared mobility solutions, such as car sharing and bike sharing services, to reduce congestion and pollution.

Information and Communication Technologies (ICT)
- **Green IT:** ICT companies are developing solutions to reduce the energy consumption of data centres and computing devices.
- **Sustainable Applications and Platforms:** Developing applications and platforms that facilitate sustainable practices, such as tracking energy consumption or sharing resources.

Sustainable Resource Management
- **Recycling and Reuse:** Companies implement advanced recycling systems and reuse initiatives to minimise waste.
- **Sustainable Water Management:** Development of technologies for more efficient use of water and for the treatment and reuse of wastewater.

Sustainable Agriculture and Food
- **Precision Agriculture:** Using technologies such as drones, sensors and artificial intelligence to optimise the use of resources in agriculture.
- **Sustainable food:** Food companies are investing in sustainable food production, including plant-based alternatives and organic production methods.

Ecological Products and Services
- **Eco-design:** Designing products that are not only efficient and useful, but also environmentally friendly and easy to recycle or break down.
- **Services based on the Circular Economy:** Creation of business models that encourage the reuse and reduction of waste.

Corporate Social Responsibility (CSR)
- **CSR programmes:** Companies are implementing CSR programmes that focus on environmental sustainability, community support and ethical working practices.

These innovations show that the private sector can be a powerful driver of sustainable change, contributing to both environmental protection and long-term economic goals. By integrating sustainability into their business models, companies can play a key role in building a more sustainable future.

Chapter 18

ENVIRONMENTAL POLICY AND GOVERNANCE

Analysis of Effective Environmental Policies

Analysing the effectiveness of environmental policies requires an assessment of the strategies and actions implemented to protect the environment and promote sustainability. Effective policies are those that achieve their objectives while being economically viable and socially acceptable. Here are some key aspects of analysing effective environmental policies:

Clear and measurable objectives
- **Definition of Objectives:** Effective policies have clear objectives, such as reducing CO_2 emissions, improving air quality or conserving biodiversity.
- **Performance Indicators:** Measurable indicators are used to assess the progress and effectiveness of policies.

Scientific Integration and Research
- **Scientific foundation:** Policies must be based on sound scientific evidence, with a clear understanding of the environmental problems they aim to solve.
- **Innovation and Adaptation:** Policies must encourage technological innovation and be flexible enough to adapt to new discoveries and changing environmental conditions.

Public Participation and Support
- **Stakeholder engagement:** Involving communities, businesses and environmental groups in policy development ensures wider understanding and support.
- **Awareness-raising and education:** Informing and educating the public about environmental issues is crucial to the success of policies.

International Cooperation
- **International agreements and standards:** Cross-border environmental problems require international cooperation, as illustrated by the Paris Climate Agreement.
- **Sharing best practice:** Exchanging information and strategies between countries can improve the effectiveness of environmental policies.

Ongoing Assessment and Review
- **Monitoring and Reporting:** Regular monitoring and transparent reporting on the results of policies help to assess their effectiveness.

- **Performance-based reviews:** Policies must be reviewed and adjusted in the light of their performance and changes in environmental and economic conditions.

Economic sustainability

- **Economic incentives:** Incentives such as subsidies for green technologies or pollution taxes can encourage sustainable practices.
- **Cost-benefit analysis:** Policies must be economically viable, with benefits that outweigh the associated costs.

Equity and Environmental Justice

- **Consideration of Vulnerable Populations:** Policies must take account of the impact on the most vulnerable populations and aim to reduce environmental inequalities.
- **Equitable Distribution of Resources:** Ensuring a fair and equitable distribution of natural resources and environmental burdens.

Analysis of effective environmental policies reveals that success depends on a combination of scientific rigour, public support, economic viability and international cooperation. A holistic and integrated approach is needed to effectively address contemporary environmental challenges.

The role of international agreements and Cooperation

International agreements and cooperation play an essential role in managing global environmental challenges such as climate change, biodiversity loss and pollution. These agreements enable nations to collaborate on strategies and actions that go beyond individual capacities and jurisdictions. Here are some key aspects of their role:

Setting Common Standards and Objectives

- **Climate agreements:** Agreements such as the Paris Climate Agreement set global targets for reducing greenhouse gas emissions and limiting global warming.
- **Protecting biodiversity:** The Convention on Biological Diversity promotes the conservation of biodiversity and the sustainable use of natural resources.

Sharing resources and knowledge
- **Technology and expertise:** International cooperation facilitates the sharing of environmentally-friendly technologies and scientific knowledge between developed and developing countries.
- **Financial assistance:** Wealthier countries often commit to providing financial support to developing countries to help them achieve their environmental objectives.

Monitoring and Reporting
- **Monitoring progress:** International agreements imply monitoring mechanisms to track countries' progress towards agreed targets.
- **Accountability and Transparency:** The need for regular reporting encourages accountability and transparency in countries' actions.

Conflict Resolution and Cross-Border Cooperation
- **Management of shared resources:** International agreements help to manage shared resources, such as river basins and transboundary ecosystems, in a sustainable and equitable way.
- **Conflict Prevention and Resolution:** They provide a framework for the prevention and resolution of conflicts related to natural resources and the environment.

Raising awareness and global commitment
- **Global awareness:** International agreements raise awareness of global environmental issues, highlighting their importance and urgency.
- **Mobilising citizens:** They can also stimulate the commitment and action of citizens, businesses and non-governmental organisations.

Adaptation and Mitigation of Environmental Effects
- **Adaptation strategies:** Countries are working together to develop strategies to adapt to the effects of climate change, such as rising sea levels and extreme weather events.
- **Disaster Risk Reduction:** International agreements can also include initiatives to reduce the risk of natural disasters and respond to environmental emergencies.

International cooperation through agreements and joint initiatives is essential to meet global environmental challenges. It enables coordinated action, reinforces global responsibility and promotes an equitable sharing of responsibilities and resources to protect our planet.

Urban Management and Planning to Reduce Pollution

Urban management and planning play a crucial role in reducing pollution. As centres of dense human activity, cities are often confronted with high levels of air, noise and water pollution. Effective urban planning can mitigate these problems while improving the quality of life of city dwellers. Here are some key strategies:

Integrated Urban Planning
- **Zoning and Land Use:** Intelligent urban planning that integrates well-planned residential, commercial and industrial zones can reduce the need for long journeys and, consequently, transport-related pollution.
- **Green spaces and blue infrastructure:** The creation of parks, gardens, green roofs and blue corridors (bodies of water) can improve air quality and provide spaces for relaxation, while helping to manage rainwater.

Sustainable transport
- **Public transport networks:** Developing efficient public transport systems, such as buses, trams and metros, to reduce dependence on private vehicles.
- **Infrastructure for cyclists and pedestrians:** Create cycle paths and wide pavements to encourage walking and cycling, thereby reducing pollution and improving public health.

Green Buildings and Energy
- **Sustainable Construction Standards:** Imposing high standards for energy efficiency and the use of sustainable materials in new buildings and renovations.
- **Renewable energy:** Promoting the use of renewable energy sources, such as solar panels and geothermal heating systems, in urban buildings.

Waste Management
- **Recycling and composting systems: Implementing** effective waste management systems to reduce the amount of waste sent to landfill and the resulting pollution.

- **Reducing waste at source:** Encouraging waste reduction practices, such as the use of reusable materials and composting.

Air Quality and Pollution Monitoring

- **Pollution Sensors:** Install sensors to monitor air quality and identify sources of pollution.
- **Emissions regulations :** Apply strict regulations on industrial and vehicle emissions to control sources of air pollution.

Raising awareness and civic participation

- **Educational programmes:** Raising public awareness of pollution problems and eco-responsible behaviour.
- **Community Involvement:** Involving residents in urban planning and green initiatives.

Urban management and planning to reduce pollution requires a holistic approach that integrates environmental, social and economic dimensions. By adopting sustainable strategies, cities can become healthier, more resilient and more pleasant places to live.

Chapter 19

ACTIVISM AND CIVIL MOBILISATION

Citizen movements and their impact

Citizens' movements have a profound impact on raising awareness and taking action on environmental and public health issues such as pollution and cancer. These movements can take many forms, from local protests to global campaigns, and they play several key roles:

Awareness-raising and education
- **Disseminating information:** Citizen movements raise public awareness of specific issues that are often neglected or underestimated by the traditional media or governments.
- **Educational Programmes:** They organise workshops, seminars and educational campaigns to inform people about environmental and health problems and how to combat them.

Pressure on political decision-makers
- **Influencing policy:** Citizens' movements can exert significant pressure on politicians to adopt or modify environmental and health policies.
- **Defending rights:** They actively defend citizens' rights to a healthy environment and access to healthcare.

Changing Social Norms
- **Behaviour change:** By raising awareness and educating, these movements can change individual and collective behaviour in favour of more sustainable and healthier practices.
- **Creating a Culture of Sustainability:** They help to establish a culture of environmental responsibility and public health awareness.

Collective Mobilisation and Action
- **Campaigns and demonstrations:** Movements organise campaigns, demonstrations and rallies to draw attention to specific issues and push for action.
- **Community participation:** They encourage the active participation of citizens in the management of their environment and the promotion of public health.

Collaboration and Networks
- **Partnerships:** Citizens' movements often work with NGOs, experts, businesses and other stakeholders to strengthen their impact.

- **Global networks:** They can connect and collaborate with similar movements internationally, sharing resources, knowledge and strategies.

Innovation and Creative Solutions
- **Development of Solutions:** These movements encourage innovation and the development of new and creative solutions to environmental and health problems.
- **Pilot projects:** They can launch pilot projects to demonstrate the effectiveness of certain practices or technologies.

Citizen movements play a vital role in promoting positive change in environmental and public health issues. By mobilising civil society, exerting political pressure and encouraging the adoption of sustainable practices, they make a significant contribution to creating a healthier and more sustainable future.

Successful collective actions

Collective action by communities, organisations or citizens' movements has led to numerous success stories in the fight against pollution and the promotion of environmental health. These actions show how collaboration and commitment can lead to significant change. Here are a few outstanding examples:

Cleaning and restoration of watercourses
- **Example:** Community initiatives to clean up and restore polluted rivers and lakes.
- **Impact:** These actions have often led to a significant improvement in water quality, benefiting both the aquatic ecosystem and local communities.

Campaigns against illegal landfill
- **Example:** Citizens' movements have organised to oppose the creation of illegal landfill sites or the establishment of polluting industries in their communities.
- **Result:** these campaigns have often succeeded in halting or relocating projects that are harmful to the environment and public health.

Reforestation and Conservation Initiatives
- **Example:** Community groups and NGOs have launched reforestation and conservation projects in degraded areas.

- **Benefits:** These initiatives have contributed to the restoration of biodiversity, carbon sequestration and soil regeneration.

Mobilisation for Environmental Policies

- **Example:** Demonstrations and petitions organised by citizens to demand stricter environmental policies.
- **Consequences:** These efforts have sometimes led to the adoption of new environmental legislation or the implementation of stricter regulations.

Development of Local Sustainable Solutions

- **Example:** Communities creating sustainable solutions, such as community waste management systems or renewable energy projects.
- **Impact:** These projects have helped to reduce dependence on fossil fuels and promote more efficient waste management.

Collective actions against large companies

- **Example:** Citizens' movements have been formed to hold big business responsible for pollution and environmental damage.
- **Results:** These actions have often led to changes in company practices, compensation for damage caused and greater awareness of the environmental impact of industrial activities.

These examples show that collective action can have a considerable impact on improving the environment and public health. They underline the importance of civic engagement and community participation in tackling environmental problems.

Strategies for Effective Participation

For effective participation in environmental or public health efforts, it is crucial to adopt strategies that encourage commitment, collaboration and action. Here are some key strategies for effective participation:

Awareness-raising and education

- **Accessible information:** Providing clear and accessible information on environmental and health issues, and on how individuals can contribute.

- **Educational Programmes:** Organising workshops, seminars and educational campaigns in schools, universities and communities to raise awareness and educate.

Encouraging community involvement

- **Local groups:** Support the formation of local groups or committees that can take action on specific issues in their community.
- **Participatory projects:** Encouraging participation in community projects such as neighbourhood clean-ups, tree planting or recycling initiatives.

Collaboration Platforms

- **Online forums:** Using online platforms to connect people, share ideas and resources, and coordinate actions.
- **Social networks:** Using social media to raise awareness, share success stories and mobilise people around environmental initiatives.

Involvement in decision-making

- **Public consultations:** Giving citizens the opportunity to take part in public consultations on environmental and health policies.
- **Working groups:** Include community representatives in working groups or advisory committees on environmental and health issues.

Volunteering and Opportunities for Action

- **Volunteer programmes:** Creating volunteer opportunities for individuals to get actively involved in environmental or public health projects.
- **Action Days:** Organise days dedicated to specific actions, such as clean-up days or cancer screening campaigns.

Recognition and incentives

- **Rewards and Recognition:** Recognising and rewarding individual or collective contributions to encourage ongoing participation.
- **Incentives:** Offer incentives, such as tax reductions or subsidies, to encourage sustainable practices within businesses and households.

Partnerships and collaboration

- **Intersectoral collaboration:** Building partnerships between governments, NGOs, businesses and community groups to tackle problems holistically.

- **Multi-Stakeholder Projects:** Involving various stakeholders in the development and implementation of environmental or health projects.

By adopting these strategies, organisations and communities can encourage active and meaningful participation, which is essential to effectively address environmental and public health challenges. Effective participation requires ongoing commitment, transparency and open communication to ensure that actions are inclusive and effective.

Chapter 20

ECONOMIC ANALYSIS POLLUTION AND CANCER

Economic Cost of Cancer and Pollution

The economic cost of cancer and pollution is substantial and multifaceted, affecting not only healthcare systems but also the global economy through lost productivity, healthcare expenditure and environmental impacts. Here is an analysis of these costs:

Direct Health Costs
- **Medical treatment:** The cost of treating cancer, including surgery, chemotherapy, radiotherapy and drugs, represents a significant proportion of healthcare expenditure.
- **Long-term care:** Cancer patients may require long-term care, increasing costs for healthcare systems and insurers.

Indirect costs linked to loss of productivity
- **Inability to work:** Cancer patients may be unable to work during their treatment and convalescence, reducing productivity and income.
- **Informal care:** Family members caring for cancer patients may have to reduce their working hours or quit their jobs.

Costs associated with pollution
- **Public health expenditure:** Air, water and soil pollution lead to increased public health costs due to the rise in respiratory, cardiovascular and cancer diseases.
- **Decontamination and clean-up:** The costs of decontaminating polluted sites and managing toxic waste are also significant.

Impact on Quality of Life
- **Deterioration in quality of life: In** addition to the financial costs, cancer and pollution have a negative impact on the quality of life of patients and the communities affected.

Costs for employers
- **Absenteeism and presenteeism:** Employers incur costs linked to the absenteeism of sick employees and presenteeism (employees working while sick, with reduced productivity).

Environmental costs
- **Loss of Biodiversity:** Pollution can lead to the loss of biodiversity, which has an economic cost, particularly in industries dependent on natural ecosystems, such as fishing and tourism.
- **Climate change:** The effects of climate change, exacerbated by pollution, are leading to additional costs in

terms of natural disasters, changes in agricultural practices and water resource management.

Socio-economic costs

- **Inequalities:** Cancer and pollution tend to affect low-income populations disproportionately, exacerbating socio-economic inequalities.
- **Government spending:** Governments must allocate significant resources to public health management, pollution regulation and prevention initiatives.

In short, cancer and pollution have considerable economic repercussions that extend beyond immediate health costs. An integrated approach combining prevention, technological innovation and public policy is needed to reduce these costs and promote a healthier, more sustainable society.

Investment in public health and Ecology

Investments in public health and ecology are essential to creating healthier, more sustainable and resilient societies. These investments can take many forms and have positive long-term impacts. Here are some key areas where such investment is crucial:

Public health infrastructure

- **Health systems:** Investing in health infrastructure, including hospitals, clinics and laboratories, to improve access to care and the capacity to respond to health emergencies.
- **Medical training:** Financing the training and development of healthcare professionals to ensure a qualified and sufficient workforce.

Research and Development

- **Medical Innovation:** Funding research and development in the medical and pharmaceutical fields to discover new treatments, vaccines and healthcare technologies.
- **Ecological research:** Investing in ecological research to better understand and preserve ecosystems, biodiversity and natural resources.

Prevention and Health Education
- **Prevention programmes:** Financing disease prevention programmes, in particular vaccination campaigns, cancer screening and the promotion of healthy lifestyles.
- **Health education:** Investing in health education to raise public awareness of health issues and encourage responsible behaviour.

Green and Sustainable Technologies
- **Renewable energies:** Supporting the development and implementation of renewable energy technologies to reduce dependence on fossil fuels and cut greenhouse gas emissions.
- **Sustainable infrastructure:** investing in sustainable urban infrastructure, including public transport, green buildings and waste management systems.

Natural Resources Management
- **Water and Soil Conservation:** Financing water and soil conservation projects to preserve these essential resources and promote their sustainable use.
- **Protecting biodiversity:** Investing in the protection of natural habitats and endangered species to maintain biodiversity.

Policies and regulations
- **Environmental and Health Legislation:** Supporting the development and implementation of policies and regulations to protect public health and the environment.
- **Standards and Incentives:** Establish environmental and health standards and provide incentives to encourage sustainable practices in the private sector.

Global Health and International Cooperation
- **International Aid:** Contributing to global health initiatives, particularly in low-income countries, to combat cross-border diseases and improve global health conditions.
- **Global Partnerships:** Working with international organisations and NGOs to promote health and sustainability on a global scale.

These investments require a coordinated approach involving governments, the private sector, non-governmental organisations and civil society. By allocating adequate resources to public health and ecology, societies can not only improve the quality of life of their citizens, but also ensure a sustainable future for generations to come.

Business Models for Sustainable Development

Economic models for sustainable development seek to balance economic growth with environmental protection and social well-being. These models aim to create value in a sustainable way, taking into account environmental and social impacts. Here are some key economic models promoting sustainable development:

Circular Economy
- **Reuse and Recycling:** Maximising the use of resources by reusing, repairing and recycling products to reduce waste.
- **Sustainable design:** designing products so that they can be easily dismantled and recycled, thereby extending their life cycle.

Green Economy
- **Investment in Green Technologies:** Direct investment towards technologies and industries that reduce environmental impact, such as renewable energies and energy efficiency.
- **Creating Green Jobs:** Developing the labour market in sectors that contribute to environmental protection.

Corporate Social Responsibility (CSR)
- **Ethical Business Practices:** Integrating social and environmental responsibility into business practices, going beyond legal compliance.
- **Community involvement:** Contributing to the economic and social development of the communities in which our businesses operate.

Socially Responsible Investment (SRI)
- **ESG criteria:** Invest in companies that respect environmental, social and governance (ESG) criteria.
- **Sustainable Development Funds:** Create specific funds to invest in projects and companies that promote sustainable development.

Blue Economy
- **Sustainable Management of Aquatic Resources:** sustainably exploiting oceans, seas and waterways for fishing, tourism and transport, while protecting aquatic ecosystems.
- **Innovation in Marine Technologies:** Developing innovative technologies for the sustainable exploitation of marine resources.

Sustainable Agriculture and Food

- **Organic and Precision Farming:** Farming that minimises environmental impact and maximises resource efficiency.
- **Local Food Systems:** Promoting local and sustainable food systems to reduce the carbon footprint of food products.

Sustainable Consumption Models

- **Responsible consumption:** Encouraging consumers to opt for sustainable products and services and to reduce their overall consumption.
- **Renting and Sharing:** Encouraging economic models based on sharing and renting rather than owning, thereby reducing the consumption of resources.

These economic models show that sustainable development can be integrated into various economic sectors. They require close collaboration between governments, businesses, consumers and other players in society if they are to succeed. By adopting these models, it is possible to promote economic growth that respects the environment and improves social well-being.

Chapter 21

THE ROLE OF EDUCATION AND TRAINING

Integration of Environmental Health in Educational Programmes

Integrating environmental health into educational programmes is crucial to developing a deeper awareness and understanding of the links between the environment, human health and well-being. Here are some key strategies for successful integration:

Curriculum Vitae
- **Educational content:** Integrating environmental health topics into school curricula at different levels, including biology, chemistry, geography and social sciences.
- **Interdisciplinary approach:** Use an interdisciplinary approach to teach how environmental issues such as pollution, climate change and biodiversity affect human health.

Practical Activities and Projects
- **Fieldwork:** Organising educational excursions to observe the environmental impacts on health in the local community.
- **Research projects:** Encourage students to carry out research projects on subjects related to environmental health.

Awareness-raising and campaigns
- **Theme Days:** Celebrate global days such as Earth Day or World Health Day to raise awareness of specific environmental health issues.
- **Awareness campaigns:** Organise campaigns in schools and universities to promote healthy, environmentally-friendly behaviour.

Teacher and trainer training
- **Professional development:** Offering training and workshops to teachers on environmental health so that they can effectively integrate this subject into their teaching.
- **Educational resources:** Providing teachers with educational resources and course materials on environmental health.

Working with experts and institutions
- **Partnerships:** Establish partnerships with universities, research bodies and NGOs to enrich educational programmes with expert knowledge and experience.

- **Guest speakers:** Invite health professionals, scientists and environmental activists to speak to the students.

Use of Educational Technologies

- **Digital tools:** Using digital tools and online platforms to teach environmental health concepts interactively.
- **Educational games:** Develop games and simulations to help students understand the complex impacts of pollution and other environmental factors on health.

Inclusive and Global Education

- **Global perspectives:** Include case studies and examples from various regions of the world to show the global and interconnected impact of environmental health.
- **Education for All:** Ensuring that environmental health education is accessible to all students, regardless of their socio-economic background.

By integrating environmental health into education, students can acquire the knowledge, skills and attitudes they need to become responsible, informed citizens capable of making informed decisions about their health and the environment.

Professional Training and Risk Awareness

Professional training and risk awareness are essential to prepare individuals to identify, understand and effectively manage risks, particularly in contexts where health, safety and the environment are at stake. Here are some key strategies for effective training and awareness-raising:

Sector-specific training programmes

- **Tailored training:** offering training programmes specific to different sectors, such as industry, health, construction and agriculture, to address the risks relevant to each area.
- **Practical training:** Include practical components in the training, such as simulations and field exercises, to better prepare participants to deal with real-life situations.

Risk awareness and prevention

- **Risk training:** Educating employees about the types of risks to which they could be exposed, including physical, chemical, biological and environmental risks.
- **Accident Prevention:** Teaching accident prevention strategies and best practices to minimise risks.

Use of Educational Technologies

- **Digital tools:** Using educational technologies such as virtual reality and e-learning to provide an immersive and interactive learning experience.
- **Online platforms:** offering online training to make learning about environmental health and safety more accessible.

Ongoing training and updates

- **Ongoing training:** Ensuring that training is ongoing and regularly updated to reflect the latest standards, technologies and methods.
- **Refresher courses:** Organise refresher courses to keep employees up to date with best practice and regulatory developments.

Raising awareness of safety culture

- **Safety Culture:** Encouraging the development of a safety culture within organisations, where health and safety are integrated into all activities.
- **Management commitment:** Involve management in training to demonstrate the company's commitment to health and safety.

Working with experts

- **External stakeholders:** Bringing in health and safety experts, regulators and industry professionals to share knowledge and experience.
- **Partnerships with institutions:** Working with universities, research institutes and professional organisations to enhance the content of the training.

Assessments and Feedback

- **Risk Assessments:** Training employees to carry out risk assessments and develop risk management plans.
- **Feedback and Improvement:** Gathering feedback on training courses to improve them and adapt them to participants' needs.

Professional training and risk awareness are fundamental to ensuring the safety and well-being of employees and to promoting sustainable and environmentally friendly working practices. A proactive and well-informed approach is essential for effective risk management in all business sectors.

Skills Development
for Prevention and Management

Developing skills in the prevention and management of environmental and health risks is crucial in the current context of growing challenges linked to climate change, pollution and public health.
Here are some key strategies for developing these skills:

Awareness-raising and education
- **Basic training:** Providing basic training on environmental and health risks, including an understanding of causes, impacts and prevention methods.
- **Specialised educational programmes:** integrating these subjects into educational programmes at all levels, from primary schools to universities.

Risk Assessment Skills
- **Risk Analysis:** Training individuals to assess environmental and health risks systematically, using scientific and statistical methods.
- **Risk Factor Identification:** Learn to identify potential risk factors in different environments, such as workplaces, communities and natural ecosystems.

Risk Management Training
- **Risk Management Planning:** Developing the skills to create and implement effective risk management plans.
- **Crisis Management:** Training in crisis management to learn how to react effectively in the event of an environmental or health emergency.

Communication skills
- **Effective communication:** Learning how to communicate risks and preventive measures clearly to the public, stakeholders and teams.
- **Raising public awareness:** Developing skills to raise public awareness of environmental and health risks and the importance of prevention.

Leadership and decision-making training
- **Informed decision-making:** Strengthening decision-making capabilities based on scientific evidence and risk analysis.

- **Safety Leadership:** Cultivating leadership skills to guide teams and communities in implementing safe and sustainable practices.

Use of Technology

- **Monitoring Technologies:** Training in the use of modern technologies to monitor and analyse environmental and health risks.
- **Digital tools:** Using digital tools for data collection, risk analysis and information dissemination.

Continuous learning and adaptability

- **Updating knowledge:** Encouraging continuous learning to keep up to date with the latest research, trends and innovations in environmental health.
- **Adaptability:** Developing the ability to adapt in order to respond effectively to new challenges and risk scenarios.

Developing these skills is essential for professionals, decision-makers, educators and the general public. By strengthening individual and collective capacities, it is possible to better prevent and manage environmental and health risks, thus contributing to safer and more resilient communities.

Chapter 22

EMERGING TECHNOLOGIES AND THEIR POTENTIAL

Biotechnology and Nanotechnology in the fight against cancer

Biotechnology and nanotechnology are playing a revolutionary role in the fight against cancer, offering innovative approaches to the diagnosis, treatment and prevention of this disease. These technologies have the potential to significantly improve the effectiveness of cancer treatments while reducing their side effects. Key areas of application include

Biotechnology in Cancer Treatment
- **Targeted therapies:** Biotechnology has enabled the development of targeted therapies that specifically attack cancer cells without damaging healthy tissue, thereby reducing side effects.
- **Immunotherapy:** Innovative techniques that stimulate or restore the immune system's ability to fight cancer, including the use of monoclonal antibodies and modified T cells.

Nanotechnology in the fight against cancer
- **Drug delivery:** Nanoparticles can be used to target and deliver anti-cancer drugs directly to tumour cells, increasing treatment efficacy and minimising exposure of healthy tissue.
- **Diagnostics and Imaging:** Nanotechnologies are improving imaging and diagnostic techniques, enabling earlier and more accurate detection of cancers.

Research and Development
- **Drug discovery:** Biotechnology facilitates the discovery and development of new cancer drugs using methods such as high-throughput screening and genomics.
- **Toxicity and side-effect studies:** Nanotechnology technologies are helping to study in detail the toxicity and potential side-effects of anti-cancer treatments.

Gene and Cell Therapy
- **Genetic modification:** Gene therapies involving the modification of the DNA of cancer cells or the patient's own immune cells offer new possibilities for treating cancer.
- **Cellular therapies:** advanced techniques using cells modified or treated in the laboratory to target and destroy cancer cells.

Customising treatments
- **Personalised medicine:** Using genetic and molecular data to develop personalised treatments based on the specific characteristics of an individual's cancer.
- **Biomarkers:** Development of biomarkers for accurate assessment of response to treatment and cancer follow-up.

Interdisciplinary collaboration
- **Cross-disciplinary collaboration:** Combining biotechnology and nanotechnology with other fields, such as computer science and engineering, to create integrated approaches in the fight against cancer.

The integration of biotechnology and nanotechnology in the fight against cancer is a promising and rapidly evolving field. These technologies bring new perspectives to the understanding and treatment of cancer, paving the way for more effective and less invasive therapies.

Pollution Reduction Technologies

Pollution abatement technologies play a crucial role in combating environmental contamination and protecting public health. Various innovations and technical developments are being deployed to tackle different types of pollution. Here are some of these technologies:

For the Reduction of Air Pollution
- **Particulate filters:** Used in industry and vehicles to trap fine particles and prevent them from being emitted into the atmosphere.
- **Scrubbers:** Industrial installations that remove gaseous pollutants, such as sulphur dioxide, from exhaust gases.
- **Catalysts:** Convert harmful vehicle exhaust gases, such as carbon monoxide, into less polluting gases.

Water Quality Technologies
- **Wastewater Treatment Systems:** Advanced technologies to treat wastewater before it is discharged into watercourses, removing excessive contaminants and nutrients.

- **Filtration and Disinfection:** Use of sand filters, activated carbon and disinfection methods such as ozonation and ultraviolet to purify the water.

Solid Waste Management

- **Recycling and Composting:** Technologies for sorting, treating and recycling waste, thereby reducing the amount of waste sent to landfill sites.
- **Incineration with Energy Recovery:** Burning waste to produce energy while reducing the volume of waste.

Noise Reduction

- **Sound Absorbing Materials:** Use of special materials in construction to absorb noise and reduce noise pollution.
- **Quiet Zones:** Creation of urban areas where traffic is limited or banned to reduce noise.

Green Technologies in Construction

- **Green Buildings:** Design and construction of buildings that use less energy, water and materials, thereby reducing their environmental impact.
- **Green Roofs and Green Walls:** Using vegetation in buildings to improve insulation, absorb CO_2 and filter pollutants.

Renewable Energy

- **Solar and Wind Energy Systems:** Deploying technologies to capture energy from the sun and wind, reducing dependence on polluting fossil fuels.
- **Biofuels:** Production of fuels from biological sources, considered cleaner and more sustainable than fossil fuels.

Electric and Hybrid Vehicles

- **Reducing exhaust gas emissions:** Adoption of electric and hybrid vehicles to reduce greenhouse gas emissions and atmospheric pollutants.

By combining these technologies with effective environmental policies and increased awareness, it is possible to significantly reduce pollution in its various forms, thereby contributing to a healthier, more sustainable environment.

Innovations in Environmental Monitoring

Innovations in environmental monitoring are essential for detecting, analysing and responding effectively to environmental problems. Advances in technology have made it possible to develop new tools and methods for monitoring the state of our environment more accurately and in real time. Here are some of these innovations:

Sensors and Monitoring Networks
- **Environmental Sensors:** Advanced sensors can measure a variety of environmental parameters such as air quality, water pollution, noise levels and radiation.
- **Monitoring networks:** Large-scale sensor networks provide real-time data on the state of the environment.

Satellite imagery and remote sensing
- **Environmental satellites:** Satellites equipped with specialised sensors can monitor vast areas for phenomena such as deforestation, changes in glaciers and atmospheric pollution.
- **Remote Sensing Data Analysis:** The use of remote sensing techniques to analyse satellite data and provide information on environmental changes on a global scale.

Drones and Unmanned Aerial Vehicles (UAVs)
- **Drones for Surveillance:** Drones are used to collect data in hard-to-reach areas, for monitoring water quality, forest health and detecting pollutants.
- **Flexibility and accessibility:** drones offer a flexible and less expensive method of collecting accurate environmental data.

Artificial Intelligence (AI) and Data Analysis
- **Processing Large Quantities of Data:** AI and machine learning can be used to analyse large quantities of environmental data to identify trends and patterns.
- **Forecasting and Modelling:** Using AI to model and forecast environmental phenomena, such as atmospheric pollution episodes and climate change.

Citizen Scientist Networks
- **Public participation:** Applications and online platforms enable citizens to contribute to environmental monitoring by sharing observations and measurements.
- **Strengthening Community Monitoring:** These networks provide more extensive baseline monitoring and involve the public in protecting the environment.

Biotechnology
- **Biomonitoring:** Use of bio-indicators, such as plants or micro-organisms, to monitor changes in the environment or the presence of pollutants.

*   **Biosensors:** Development of biosensors sensitive to certain types of pollutants or environmental conditions.

Connectivity and Data Integration

*   **Integrated systems:** Integration of different data sources for a complete picture of the state of the environment.
*   **Accessible Platforms:** Development of platforms where environmental data is easily accessible to researchers, decision-makers and the public.

These innovations improve our ability to monitor, understand and respond to environmental challenges. They are crucial to effective environmental management and informed decision-making in the fight against pollution and climate change.

Chapter 23

LEGAL AND REGULATORY ASPECTS

International and national legislation

International and national legislation plays a crucial role in managing and protecting the environment and promoting public health. These laws and regulations provide the framework needed to address environmental and health challenges on a global and local scale. Here are some key aspects of international and national legislation:

International legislation
- **Environmental Agreements and Treaties:** Agreements such as the Paris Climate Agreement, the Convention on Biological Diversity, and the Montreal Protocol on Substances that Deplete the Ozone Layer aim to address global environmental issues.
- **International standards and directives:** International organisations such as the World Health Organisation (WHO) and the United Nations (UN) set standards and directives to guide environmental and health policies.

National legislation
- **Environmental protection laws:** Countries adopt national laws to regulate polluting emissions, manage waste, protect natural resources and conserve biodiversity.
- **Public health regulations:** National legislation also includes regulations on drinking water quality, the management of toxic substances and public health monitoring.

Implementation and Compliance
- **Enforcement:** National governments are responsible for enforcing environmental and health laws through regulatory agencies and monitoring programmes.
- **Penalties and incentives:** Legislation often provides penalties for non-compliance as well as incentives to encourage sustainable and sound practices.

Stakeholder participation and involvement
- **Public consultation:** Legislation is often drafted with the participation of stakeholders, including NGOs, businesses, experts and the public.
- **Cross-border cooperation:** Cross-border environmental problems require cooperation and legislative coordination between neighbouring countries.

Adaptation and Evolution of Laws
- **Regular Reviews:** Environmental and health laws must be regularly reviewed to adapt to new scientific discoveries, technological innovations and changing environmental challenges.
- **Reactive legislation:** Ability to respond rapidly to environmental and health emergencies with appropriate legislative measures.

Harmonisation of laws
- **Harmonisation with International Standards:** Countries often strive to harmonise their national legislation with international agreements and standards to ensure global consistency.

By combining efforts at international and national level, legislation can effectively address environmental and health challenges. This requires ongoing cooperation, adaptation to change and the active involvement of all stakeholders.

Environmental and Health Law

Environmental and health law is an important branch of law that focuses on laws and regulations designed to protect the environment and promote public health. It covers a wide range of areas, including air and water quality, waste management, biodiversity conservation, and the control of hazardous chemicals. Here are some key aspects of environmental and health law:

Air Quality Laws and Regulations
- **Pollutant emissions :** Air quality regulations aim to control industrial emissions, vehicle emissions and other sources of air pollution.
- **Air Quality Standards:** Standards are set for key air pollutants, such as sulphur dioxide, nitrogen oxides and fine particles.

Water and Water Quality Management
- **Surface and ground water:** Laws regulate the pollution of surface and ground water, and set standards for drinking water quality.

- **Wastewater management:** Regulations on the treatment and discharge of industrial and municipal wastewater to protect aquatic ecosystems.

Waste and toxic substances management

- **Waste disposal:** Legislation governs the collection, treatment and disposal of solid waste, including hazardous waste.
- **Control of Chemical Substances:** Regulations on the use, storage and transport of hazardous chemical substances to prevent harmful exposure.

Biodiversity conservation

- **Protection of Species and Habitats:** Laws designed to protect endangered species and their habitats, as well as regulating the use of natural resources.
- **International agreements:** Participation in international agreements such as the Convention on International Trade in Endangered Species of Wild Fauna and Flora (CITES).

Public Health and Food Safety

- **Public Health Standards:** Regulations concerning public health, including disease prevention, food safety standards and health crisis management.
- **Food and Drug Product Control:** Laws governing the safety and quality of food and drug products.

International Environmental Law

- **Global Environmental Agreements:** Participation in and implementation of international agreements, such as the Paris Agreement on Climate Change and the Convention on Biological Diversity.
- **Cross-border cooperation:** Management of environmental problems that cross national borders, such as cross-border air pollution and the management of shared water resources.

Citizen Participation and Access to Information

- **Citizens' rights:** Laws guaranteeing citizens' right to environmental information, public participation in environmental decision-making processes and access to justice in environmental matters.

Environmental and health law is essential to ensure a balance between economic development and the protection of the environment and public health. It requires coordination between national and international legislation, as well as effective implementation and enforcement.

Landmark legal cases and precedents

In the field of environmental and health law, a number of legal cases have had a significant impact and set important precedents. These cases have often influenced policy, strengthened legislation and raised awareness of critical issues. Here are a few notable examples:

Industrial pollution
- **Love Canal case:** In the 1970s in the United States, this case highlighted the dangers of industrial pollution when buried toxic chemicals began to seep into a residential area, causing serious health problems. This led to the creation of Superfund, a federal law to clean up contaminated sites.

Climate Change Litigation
- **Urgenda v Netherlands:** In 2019, the Dutch Supreme Court ruled that the Dutch government must take more ambitious measures to reduce greenhouse gas emissions, setting a precedent for government responsibility for climate change.

Legal action against polluting companies
- **Trial against Chevron in Ecuador:** A case in which Chevron was ordered to pay billions of dollars for environmental contamination in the Ecuadorian Amazon. Although controversial and complicated by international legal issues, the case drew attention to corporate responsibility for pollution.

Rights of indigenous communities
- **Case of Ogoniland in Nigeria:** Ogoni communities have taken legal action against Shell for environmental and health damage caused by oil extraction, highlighting the rights of indigenous communities and the responsibilities of multinationals.

The right to a healthy environment
- **T.C. (M.C. Mehta) v. Union of India:** India's Supreme Court has played a key role in promoting the right to a healthy environment, notably by imposing strict regulations on polluting industries.

Asbestos legislation
- **Asbestos in Europe and North America:** Legal action against asbestos manufacturers has led to major changes

in the regulation of asbestos, recognising its serious health hazards.

Protection of endangered species

- **Cases concerning the Endangered Species Act in the United States:** Several cases have strengthened this law, which protects endangered species and their habitats, influencing land management and environmental regulations.

These cases illustrate how the law can be used to address environmental and public health issues, sometimes providing the only recourse for affected communities and acting as a powerful lever for political and social change. They also highlight the complexity of environmental issues and the need for a balanced approach between economic development and environmental and public health protection.

Chapter 24

GLOBAL HEALTH AND INTERNATIONAL ISSUES

Pollution and Cancer in a Global Context

The relationship between pollution and cancer in a global context is a matter of major concern because of the significant impact of pollution on public health worldwide. Here is an analysis of this relationship:

Global Impact of Pollution
- **Air pollution:** Recognised as a major carcinogen, air pollution, especially fine particles and pollutants such as benzene, is associated with an increased risk of cancer, particularly lung cancer.
- **Water pollution:** Contamination of water sources by industrial chemicals, pesticides and heavy metals can also contribute to the incidence of various cancers.

Geographical and socio-economic disparities
- **High-risk regions:** Certain regions, particularly in developing countries where environmental regulations are weak, are more exposed to carcinogenic pollutants.
- **Health inequalities:** Low-income populations are often more exposed to pollution and have limited access to healthcare, exacerbating health inequalities.

Contributing factors
- **Industrialisation and urbanisation:** The acceleration of industrialisation and urbanisation, particularly in developing countries, has led to an increase in air and water pollution.
- **Waste management:** Inadequate management of industrial, chemical and domestic waste contributes to environmental pollution.

Research and Scientific Studies
- **Epidemiological studies:** Numerous epidemiological studies have established links between exposure to various pollutants and an increased risk of cancer.
- **Research into Mechanisms:** Research continues to explore the mechanisms by which pollutants cause damage at cellular and genetic level, leading to cancer.

Actions and Global Policies
- **International agreements:** Global efforts, such as the Paris Climate Agreement, aim to reduce emissions of greenhouse gases and other pollutants.

- **Public health initiatives:** Public health programmes aim to monitor and reduce exposure to pollutants, and to improve access to healthcare.

Awareness-raising and education

- **Public awareness: Raising** awareness of the health risks of pollution is crucial to encouraging changes in behaviour and supporting public health policies.
- **Education and training:** Education about environmental risks and cancer prevention is essential, particularly in the regions most affected.

International Cooperation and Aid

- **Assistance to developing countries:** International cooperation and aid to developing countries are needed to improve environmental management and healthcare systems.

Pollution and cancer in a global context represent a complex challenge requiring a multisectoral approach involving public health, the environment, legislation and international cooperation. A focus on prevention, research and better regulation can make a significant contribution to reducing the global burden of pollution-related cancer.

International efforts and cross-border cooperation

International efforts and cross-border cooperation are essential to effectively manage environmental and public health challenges that know no borders. These global challenges, such as climate change, pollution and the spread of disease, require a coordinated international response. Here are some key areas where this cooperation is crucial:

Climate change

- **International agreements:** The Paris Agreement is a major example of international cooperation aimed at limiting global warming by reducing greenhouse gas emissions.
- **Technology and Knowledge Sharing:** Cooperation in the research and development of low-carbon technologies and the sharing of best practices to mitigate climate change.

Preserving biodiversity
- **International conventions:** The Convention on Biological Diversity and other agreements aim to protect threatened species and habitats around the world.
- **Cross-border conservation projects:** the joint management of protected areas and ecosystems that extend beyond national borders.

Pollution Management
- **Treatment of Transboundary Pollutants:** Agreements such as the Stockholm Convention on Persistent Organic Pollutants address the management of toxic substances that move across borders.
- **Environmental Monitoring and Standards:** Cooperation in pollution monitoring and the development of international environmental standards.

Controlling infectious diseases
- **Disease surveillance:** Collaboration in surveillance and rapid response to cross-border epidemics, such as COVID-19.
- **Vaccine Research and Development:** sharing resources and knowledge to develop and distribute vaccines.

Natural Resources Management
- **Water Resource Management:** Cooperation in the management of cross-border river basins to ensure sustainable and equitable use of water.
- **Tropical Forest Conservation:** joint initiatives to conserve tropical forests, which are crucial for biodiversity and the global climate.

Sustainable development
- **Sustainable Development Goals (SDGs):** The United Nations established the SDGs to promote global sustainable development, addressing issues such as poverty, hunger, health, education, gender equality, clean water, energy and climate change.
- **International Aid and Financing :** Financial and technical assistance to developing countries to help them achieve the MDGs.

Training and Knowledge Exchange
- **Training Programmes:** Educational exchanges and training programmes to share expertise and skills in the fields of the environment and public health.

- **Research networks:** collaboration between universities and research institutes to conduct studies on global environmental and health issues.

International and cross-border cooperation is therefore essential if we are to meet global challenges in an effective and coordinated way, drawing on the diversity of experience, resources and knowledge available around the world.

Specific challenges facing developing countries

Developing countries face specific environmental and public health management challenges, often exacerbated by limited resources and economic constraints. The following is an analysis of these challenges:

Limited infrastructure and resources
- **Access to healthcare:** Limited access to quality healthcare services makes it difficult to prevent and treat illnesses, including pollution-related cancers.
- **Waste management infrastructures:** often inadequate, leading to problems of water and air pollution.

Accrus Environmental Problems
- **Industrial and urban pollution:** Rapid economic growth and urbanisation can lead to an increase in pollution without adequate environmental regulations.
- **Deforestation and Biodiversity Loss:** Major problems in many developing countries, affecting ecosystems and contributing to climate change.

Economic and social challenges
- **Poverty:** Widespread poverty limits the ability of governments and individuals to invest in sustainable health and environmental solutions.
- **Education and awareness:** Lower levels of education can limit awareness of environmental health problems and prevention practices.

Vulnerability to Climate Change
- **Impact of Climate Change:** Developing countries are often more vulnerable to the impacts of climate change, such as extreme weather events and rising sea levels.
- **Resources for Adaptation:** Lack of resources to implement effective adaptation strategies.

Dependence on Natural Resources

- **Resource-based economies:** Heavy reliance on agriculture, fishing and resource extraction, making economies and livelihoods vulnerable to environmental problems.
- **Resource management:** Challenges in the sustainable management of natural resources, exacerbated by demographic and economic pressure.

Policies and Legislation

- **Weak regulatory framework:** Environmental and public health policies and regulations are often insufficient or ineffective.
- **Corruption and governance:** Corruption and governance problems can hamper the application of environmental and health laws.

International Cooperation and Aid

- **Need for international aid:** Dependence on international aid and technical cooperation to tackle health and environmental problems.
- **Technology transfer:** Limited access to advanced technologies for environmental monitoring, disease treatment and resource management.

Efforts to overcome these challenges require an integrated approach that combines economic development, environmental protection, improved public health and education. International cooperation, investment in infrastructure and technology, and local capacity building are essential to help developing countries meet these challenges.

Chapter 25

FUTURE PERSPECTIVES AND INNOVATIONS

Future Scenarios in Function of Actual Actions

Current environmental management, public health and policy actions have a significant impact on future scenarios. Depending on whether these actions are proactive and effective or insufficient, future outcomes can vary considerably. Here is an analysis of these potential scenarios:

Optimistic scenario: Proactive and effective actions

- **Reducing greenhouse gas emissions:** If current actions are in line with the objectives of the Paris Agreement, this could limit global warming and reduce the impact of climate change.
- **Improved air and water quality:** Effective regulation and advanced technology could lead to significant improvements in air and water quality, reducing pollution-related illnesses.
- **Biodiversity conservation:** Successful efforts to conserve habitats and protect species could preserve biodiversity.
- **Strengthened public health:** Improved health systems and increased disease prevention could lead to a healthier world population.

Medium scenario: Insufficient or unequal efforts

- **Moderate Climate Change:** If action is uneven or delayed, climate change could continue at a moderate pace, leading to more frequent extreme weather events and environmental impacts.
- **Limited improvements in pollution:** Partial improvements in air and water pollution may not be enough to completely prevent pollution-related illnesses.
- **Continued Biodiversity Loss:** Without stronger conservation measures, biodiversity loss could continue, affecting ecosystems and the services they provide.
- **Persistent public health problems:** Limited progress in health systems may not completely resolve environment-related health problems.

Pessimistic scenario: Lack of Action or Ineffective Actions

- **Severe Climate Change:** Failure to take significant action on climate change could lead to major global warming, with catastrophic consequences for the environment and society.
- **Deterioration of the environment:** Continued pollution and environmental degradation could lead to more serious public health problems and a reduced quality of life.

- **Public health crises:** The lack of significant improvements in healthcare and disease prevention could lead to public health crises, particularly in low-income countries.
- **Economic and social loss:** Severe environmental and health impacts could lead to major economic losses and social instability.

These scenarios underline the importance of current actions and political decisions in shaping the future of our planet and its inhabitants. Proactive, coordinated and global action is essential if we are to move towards a more sustainable and healthier future.

The role of Research and Development

Research and development (R&D) plays a fundamental role in solving environmental and public health problems. It is essential for innovation, finding new solutions and improving existing technologies and practices. Here are some key areas where R&D is particularly crucial:

Technological Innovation
- **Development of Clean Technologies:** R&D is essential to create technologies that reduce pollution, improve energy efficiency and promote the use of renewable energies.
- **Biotechnology:** In the field of health, biotechnology offers significant advances in the treatment and prevention of diseases, including cancer.

Climate change
- **Mitigation and Adaptation:** Research helps to develop strategies for mitigating climate change and adapting to its impacts, in particular through the study of ecosystems, meteorological phenomena and climate models.
- **Carbon sequestration:** R&D is exploring methods to capture and store carbon dioxide in order to reduce greenhouse gas concentrations in the atmosphere.

Public health
- **Medical Research:** R&D is vital for discovering new medicines, vaccines and therapies to combat a range of diseases, including those linked to environmental factors.

- **Epidemiology:** Research in this field helps to understand how environmental factors affect public health and contribute to the development of diseases such as cancer.

Environmental sustainability

- **Natural Resource Management:** R&D helps to develop sustainable methods for managing water, soil and biological resources.
- **Sustainable agriculture:** Research into sustainable agricultural practices aims to increase productivity while minimising environmental impact.

Economics and Policy

- **Economic analysis:** R&D provides essential analyses for understanding the economic costs of environmental and health problems and for assessing the effectiveness of policies.
- **Policy development:** Research helps to formulate evidence-based policies to effectively manage environmental and health challenges.

Education and awareness

- **Educational programmes:** R&D helps to develop educational programmes to raise awareness and inform the public about environmental and health issues.

R&D is a driver of progress and innovation, essential to meeting the environmental and public health challenges of today and tomorrow. Investment in R&D is therefore crucial to ensuring a sustainable and healthy future.

Innovative Visions for a Healthier World

To create a healthier, more sustainable world, innovative visions are needed, combining technology, policy, education and behavioural change. Here are some ideas and concepts that could shape a healthier future:

City of the Future: Sustainable urban planning

- **Green Cities:** Designing cities that incorporate green spaces, green roofs and living walls to improve air quality and provide spaces for relaxation.
- **Sustainable mobility:** Promoting public transport, electric vehicles, cycle networks and walking to reduce air pollution and noise.

- **Energy-efficient buildings:** Constructing buildings that use renewable energy, sustainable materials and intelligent technologies to reduce energy consumption.

Health Innovation

- **Personalised medicine:** Using genetic and biomedical data to personalise treatments and disease prevention.
- **Wearable Technology:** Developing wearable devices that monitor health and encourage healthy lifestyles.
- **Telemedicine:** Using telemedicine to improve access to healthcare, particularly in remote areas.

Food and Sustainable Agriculture

- **Precision Agriculture:** Using technologies such as sensors, drones and AI to make farming more efficient and less impactful on the environment.
- **Alternative foods:** Promoting the development and consumption of sustainable foods, such as plant proteins and laboratory-grown meat.

Circular Economy

- **Zero Waste:** Moving towards a circular economy where all products are designed to be fully recyclable or biodegradable.
- **Reuse and Recycling:** Encouraging reuse and recycling to reduce waste production and resource consumption.

Renewable and Clean Energy

- **Energy Transition:** Accelerating the switch to renewable energies, such as solar, wind and hydroelectric power, to reduce dependence on fossil fuels.
- **Energy storage:** Developing efficient energy storage solutions to manage the variability of renewable energies.

Education and awareness

- **Educational programmes:** Integrate environmental and health education into all levels of education to raise awareness from an early age.
- **Awareness campaigns:** Using the media and communication campaigns to raise public awareness of environmental and health issues.

Global Cooperation

- **International partnerships:** Strengthening international cooperation to share knowledge, technologies and resources in the fight against global environmental and health problems.

These innovative visions require a multidisciplinary approach and collaboration between governments, businesses, non-governmental organisations and citizens. By embracing these ideas, we can work together to build a healthier, more sustainable future for generations to come.

Chapter 26

IN-DEPTH CONCLUSION

Summary of issues and solutions

This summary of environmental health and sustainability issues and solutions highlights the complexity of the current challenges, while highlighting possible avenues for effective solutions. Here is a summary of the main points:

Key issues
- **Climate change:** widespread effects on the environment, ecosystems and human health.
- **Pollution:** Impact on air, water and soil quality, contributing to various health problems, including cancer.
- **Biodiversity loss:** Reduction in biodiversity due to deforestation, pollution and climate change.
- **Resource degradation:** Over-exploitation of natural resources threatening environmental sustainability.
- **Social and Health Inequalities:** Disparities in the impact and management of environmental and health problems between and within countries.

Proposed Solutions
- **Transition to Renewable Energies:** Reducing dependence on fossil fuels to limit greenhouse gas emissions.
- **Technological Innovation:** Developing clean and efficient technologies to manage pollution and improve public health.
- **Policies and legislation:** Strengthening regulatory frameworks for environmental protection and health promotion.
- **International cooperation:** Working together on a global scale to tackle cross-border issues such as climate change and pollution.
- **Education and awareness:** Informing and raising public awareness of environmental and health issues to encourage sustainable behaviour.
- **Sustainable practices:** Adopting sustainable practices in agriculture, industry and everyday life to minimise environmental impact.
- **Research and Development:** Investing in research to better understand environmental and health challenges and develop new solutions.

Integration and Multidisciplinary Approach
- **Holistic approach:** Integrating environmental, economic and social considerations for a sustainable and equitable approach.
- **Multisectoral collaboration:** Involving various sectors - government, industry, civil society and the scientific community - in the search for solutions.

In summary, addressing environmental health and sustainability issues requires concerted action at all levels - local, national and international. Innovative and integrated approaches are essential to create a healthier and more sustainable future for current and future generations.

Call for Concerted Action and Multidisciplinary

Faced with the complex issues of environmental health and sustainability, a call for concerted, multidisciplinary action is crucial. This call recognises that effective solutions to these problems require collaboration between different sectors and disciplines. Here are the key elements of this call for action:

Global Collaboration
- **International partnerships:** Strengthening cooperation between nations, international organisations, NGOs and the private sector to tackle environmental and health issues that transcend borders.
- **International agreements:** Engaging in international agreements and global initiatives to tackle issues such as climate change, biodiversity loss and pollution.

Integration of Disciplines
- **Interdisciplinary approach:** Bringing together expertise from different fields, such as environmental science, medicine, engineering, economics and social sciences, to develop comprehensive solutions.
- **Research and Innovation:** Promoting interdisciplinary research and innovation to create new technologies and strategies to protect the environment and improve public health.

Political and legislative commitment
- **Strong Policies:** Adopt effective policies and legislation to regulate polluting activities, promote sustainable practices and support public health.
- **Enforcement and monitoring:** Ensuring that environmental and health laws are rigorously applied and setting up monitoring systems to assess progress.

Community contribution
- **Public Involvement:** Encouraging the active participation of local communities in decision-making and environmental initiatives.
- **Education and awareness:** Raising awareness and educating the public about environmental and health issues to encourage responsible behaviour.

Investment and Financing
- **Financial support:** Increase investment in green technologies, environmental health research and sustainable development initiatives.
- **Economic incentives: Introduce** economic incentives to encourage businesses and individuals to adopt sustainable practices.

Corporate Responsibility
- **CSR:** Encouraging companies to adopt Corporate Social Responsibility (CSR) and integrate sustainability into their business models.
- **Private Sector Innovation:** Stimulating innovation in the private sector to develop sustainable, environmentally-friendly solutions.

Adaptability and resilience
- **Adaptation plans:** Developing strategies to increase resilience to environmental and health changes, particularly in vulnerable communities.
- **Risk Management:** Strengthening environmental and health risk management to anticipate and respond effectively to crises.

This call for concerted, multidisciplinary action underlines the importance of a global, integrated approach to meeting the challenges of our time. It calls for collaboration, innovation and commitment at all levels of society to build a more sustainable and healthy future.

Additional Resources for Professionals

Practical Guides and Reference Tools

For professionals and stakeholders involved in environmental health, sustainability and sustainable development, practical guides and reference tools are essential for effective action. Here is a selection of useful resources:

Practical Guides

- **EPA (Environmental Protection Agency) guides:** The EPA provides a variety of practical guides on managing air quality, water quality, waste management and the remediation of polluted sites.
- **WHO manuals:** The World Health Organisation publishes manuals on public health, disease prevention and environmental health risk management.

Reference Tools

Environmental databases: Databases such as the Global Biodiversity Information Facility (GBIF) or the World Air Quality Index provide crucial information on various environmental parameters.

- **Environmental Atlases and Maps:** Tools such as Google Earth or the World Resources Institute's Global Forest Watch offer interactive visualisations of environmental data.

Online resources

- **Educational platforms:** Sites such as Coursera, edX and Khan Academy offer free or low-cost online courses on the environment, sustainability and public health.
- **On-line documentation:** Access reports, articles and case studies via academic publication sites such as PubMed, ScienceDirect and JSTOR.

Applications and Software

- **Environmental modelling software:** Tools such as ArcGIS for mapping and spatial analysis, or climate and environmental modelling software.
- **Mobile applications:** smartphone applications that provide real-time information on air quality, weather or carbon footprint.

Books and Publications

- **Reference books:** Reference books on ecology, environmental health and sustainable development.
- **Specialised periodicals:** Specialised newspapers and magazines offering in-depth analysis and updates on the latest research and trends.

Forums and Professional Networks

- **Discussion Groups:** Join online discussion groups, forums or professional networks to share knowledge and experience.
- **Conferences and Webinars:** Participate in conferences, seminars and webinars to keep abreast of the latest developments and best practices.

Assessment and Analysis Tools

- **Analysis kits:** Use kits and equipment to analyse water quality, air quality and other environmental parameters.
- **Checklists and Audits:** Checklists and audit guides to assess compliance with environmental and health standards.

These resources are invaluable in providing up-to-date information, best practice and strategies for effectively managing environmental and public health challenges. They are essential for professionals seeking to improve their skills, stay informed and make a significant contribution to sustainability and environmental health.

Contact Network
and Professional Collaboration

Establishing a network of contacts and professional collaborations is essential in the fields of environmental health, sustainability and sustainable development. A strong network can provide opportunities for learning, knowledge sharing, project collaboration and political influence. Here are some tips for building and maintaining an effective professional network:

Participate in conferences and professional events

- **Conferences and Seminars:** Attend national and international conferences to meet industry experts and professionals.
- **Workshops and Training :** Take part in workshops and training courses to broaden your skills and meet colleagues with similar interests.

Joining professional associations

- **Associations and organisations:** Join professional associations related to your field of specialisation to access resources, events and professional networks.
- **Working groups and committees:** Get involved in working groups or committees within these associations to work on specific issues and establish close working relationships.

Using professional social networks

- **LinkedIn:** Create and maintain a professional profile on LinkedIn to connect with professionals around the world.
- **Online groups:** Join online groups on platforms such as LinkedIn or ResearchGate to discuss topical issues and share information.

Academic and Research Collaborations

- **University partnerships:** collaborate with universities or research institutes to take part in research projects, joint publications or exchange programmes.
- **Research networks:** Join national or international research networks to collaborate on interdisciplinary projects.

Establish relations with the industrial sector and NGOs

- **Public-Private Partnerships:** Explore partnership opportunities with companies committed to sustainability and social responsibility.
- **Working with NGOs:** Collaborate with NGOs on projects, awareness campaigns or research initiatives.

Development of Joint Projects

- **Collaborative Initiatives:** Launch or join collaborative initiatives that bring together experts from different fields to tackle specific problems.
- **Sharing resources and expertise:** Exchange resources, data and expertise with your peers to enrich each other's work.

Communication and Follow-up

- **Keep in touch:** Maintain contact with your colleagues and professional acquaintances through regular updates, emails or informal meetings.
- **Mentoring:** Be a mentor to young professionals or seek mentoring to develop your career and expand your network.

By building up a solid network of contacts and collaborations, you can not only improve your professional prospects, but also make a significant contribution to collective efforts for a more sustainable and healthy future.

Conclusion

Final thoughts

Discussions on environmental health, sustainability and sustainable development underline the importance and urgency of these issues in today's world. Here are some final thoughts to take away with you:

Interconnection of Issues

- **Globality:** Environmental health and sustainability issues are interconnected and global, requiring a holistic understanding and approach.
- **Shared responsibility:** Every individual, community, business and government has a role to play in creating a more sustainable and healthy future.

The importance of collective action

- **Cooperation:** International and cross-sector cooperation is essential to effectively tackle environmental and public health challenges.
- **Community involvement:** The active participation of communities is crucial to implementing sustainable and effective solutions.

The role of Innovation and Technology

- **Technology:** Technological innovations offer powerful solutions for mitigating pollution, treating disease and managing natural resources.
- **Research:** Investment in research is essential to understanding complex problems and developing new strategies and tools.

Education and awareness

- **Knowledge:** Educating and raising awareness at all levels of society is fundamental to changing behaviour and promoting sustainable practices.
- **Training:** Ongoing training for professionals in these fields is crucial to keep up to date with the latest advances and best practices.

Vision for the future

- **Sustainability:** Adopting a long-term vision for sustainability is crucial to ensuring the health and well-being of future generations.
- **Balance:** It is important to strike a balance between economic development, environmental protection and social well-being.

In summary, the challenges of environmental health and sustainability are vast and complex, but with cooperation, innovation and shared commitment, it is possible to make progress towards a brighter future. This requires concerted action, informed decision-making and a willingness to adapt and learn continuously.

Call to Action: What can you do?

Faced with the challenges of environmental health and sustainability, everyone can contribute in their own way. Here's a call to action for everyone, highlighting concrete actions you can take:

For Individuals

- **Adopt Sustainable Practices:** Reduce your carbon footprint by favouring public transport, cycling or walking, reducing energy consumption and opting for environmentally-friendly products.
- **Education and awareness:** Find out more about environmental issues and share your knowledge with those around you.
- **Responsible consumption:** Choose sustainable products, reduce food waste and favour local and seasonal produce.

For Professionals

- **Innovation in Your Field:** Incorporate sustainable practices into your work, whether in business, research or education.
- **Networking and collaboration:** Work with colleagues and organisations to promote sustainability initiatives.

For Companies

- **Corporate Social Responsibility:** Integrate CSR into your business model, taking into account the environmental and social impacts of your activities.
- **Green Innovation:** Invest in clean technologies and sustainable practices to reduce your environmental footprint.

For decision-makers and politicians

- **Enlightened Policies:** Develop and support policies that promote sustainability, environmental protection and public health.
- **Investment in Research and Innovation:** Allocate funds for research into sustainable technologies and solving environmental problems.

For Educators and Researchers

- **Integrating sustainability into education:** teaching the principles of sustainability and environmental health in school curricula.
- **Applied Research:** Focus your research on practical solutions to environmental and health challenges.

For Communities

- **Local Initiatives:** Participate in or initiate community projects focused on sustainability, such as community gardens, recycling programmes or clean-up campaigns.

- **Community Mobilisation:** Engage your community in discussions and actions on sustainability and environmental health.

Every action, large or small, contributes to a more sustainable future. By working together, we can make a significant difference in tackling environmental challenges and promoting health and wellbeing for all.

Glossary of Technical Terms

To navigate effectively in the fields of environmental health and sustainability, it is useful to know some key technical terms. Here is a glossary of frequently used terms:

Climate change

- **Greenhouse effect: A** natural phenomenon amplified by human activities, in which certain gases in the atmosphere trap heat, leading to global warming.
- **Greenhouse gas emissions:** Gases released by human activities, such as carbon dioxide (CO_2) and methane (CH_4), which contribute to climate change.

Pollution

- **Fine particles (PM2.5) :** Tiny particles or droplets in the air that can penetrate deep into the lungs and cause health problems.
- **Persistent Organic Contaminants (POCs):** Chemical substances that are resistant to environmental degradation and can accumulate in food chains.

Environmental Health

- **Carcinogen:** Substance or agent capable of causing cancer.

- **Bioaccumulation:** Accumulation of chemical substances, such as heavy metals or pesticides, in a living organism.

Sustainability and Sustainable Development

- **Carbon footprint:** Measure of the impact of human activities on the climate in terms of the total quantity of greenhouse gases emitted.
- **Circular Economy:** Economic system designed to minimise waste and maximise the reuse and recycling of resources.

Biodiversity and Ecosystems

- **Threatened species:** Species whose population is in danger of extinction due to environmental changes or other factors.
- **Ecosystem services:** Benefits that humans derive from ecosystems, such as water purification, crop pollination and climate regulation.

Energy and Technology

- **Renewable energies:** Naturally regenerative sources of energy, such as solar, wind and hydroelectric power.
- **Biotechnology:** Use of biological systems and organisms to develop or manufacture products.

Policy and Governance

- **Sustainable development:** Development that meets the needs of the present without compromising the ability of future generations to meet their own needs.
- **Environmental regulations:** Laws and rules established to protect the environment and public health.

This glossary is not exhaustive, but it provides a basis for understanding the key terms frequently encountered in discussions on environmental health and sustainability.

Useful resources and Further Reading

To deepen your understanding of topics relating to environmental health, sustainability and sustainable development, there are many resources and further reading available. Here is a recommended selection:

Books and Publications

- **"Silent Spring" by Rachel Carson:** A classic that raised public awareness of the dangers of pesticides and stimulated the environmental movement.
- **"The Sixth Extinction" by Elizabeth Kolbert:** An exploration of past and current mass extinctions caused by human activity.
- **Reports of the Intergovernmental Panel on Climate Change (IPCC):** Provide in-depth scientific assessments of climate change.

Websites and Databases

- **World Health Organization (WHO) website:** For information on public health and environmental impacts.
- **Environmental Protection Agency (EPA) website:** resources on environmental legislation, guides to good practice and data on pollution.
- **Global Biodiversity Information Facility (GBIF):** A portal for biodiversity data from around the world.

Online courses and MOOCs

- **Coursera and edX:** offer online courses on subjects such as sustainable development, environmental management and public health.
- **Khan Academy:** Offers free educational resources on scientific and environmental subjects.

Conferences and Webinars

- **TED Talks:** inspiring talks on subjects related to the environment, science and sustainability.
- **Webinars of the International Union for Conservation of Nature (IUCN):** Discussions on biodiversity conservation and environmental policies.

Newspapers and Magazines

- **Nature and Science:** Two of the most respected scientific journals, publishing cutting-edge research in a variety of fields, including the environment and health.
- **National Geographic:** Articles and reports on the environment, science and culture.

Professional Organisations and Networks

- **World Federation of Public Health Associations (WFPHA):** A global network for public health professionals.
- **Professional networks such as LinkedIn:** Keep in touch with experts and organisations in the field of environmental health and sustainability.

Documentaries and Films

- **"An Inconvenient Truth":** A documentary on climate change, directed by former US Vice-President Al Gore.
- **"Our Planet" on Netflix:** A documentary series about the Earth's natural beauty and the impact of climate change on all living things.

These resources offer an in-depth and diverse perspective on current and future environmental and public health issues, helping to promote better understanding and more informed action.

Acknowledgements

Thank you for your commitment to learning and discussing the crucial topics of environmental health and sustainability. Your interest in these issues shows an awareness and responsibility towards our planet and its inhabitants, which is essential to bringing about positive change.

Don't forget that every effort, large or small, towards understanding and taking action in these areas contributes to a significant collective impact. Your willingness to learn, share knowledge and actively participate in these discussions is an important step towards a more sustainable and healthy future.

If you have any other questions, need further clarification or would like to explore other topics, please don't hesitate to ask. Once again, thank you for your commitment and curiosity. Keep exploring, learning and contributing to these vital topics.